The Duffy-Rath System: An Introduction

A Prevention-based Approach for Activity-related Musculoskeletal Disorders & Disability – Clinician's Edition

Wayne Rath, PT, Dip MDT
Jean Duffy Rath, PT, Dip MDT

FOREWORD

Jean and I went into clinical practice together in 1984 and incorporated as the Spine Center of New Jersey in 1985 – the same year we were married. Our first major client involved providing onsite physical therapy treatment for cumulative strain disorders in a large medical products manufacturing company. The medical director had reached out to us because of a growing problem with carpal tunnel syndrome that was not responding to their ergonomic, treatment, health and wellness programs. We successfully resolved all their cases with a novel approach, now known as the Duffy-Rath System©. All of these resistant carpal tunnel cases had a cervical source to their upper limb symptoms and dysfunction that had been previously overlooked.

During our first year onsite we identified a consistent pattern of musculoskeletal complaints and problems. The most prevalent were back and neck pain, shoulder impingement, elbow epicondylar pain, carpal tunnel syndrome, trigger finger or thumb, O/A of the basal joint of the thumb and DJD of the hip and knee. All these patients had prior warning signals but either did not recognize them or were unable to do anything effective. We educated and trained each patient to recognize and control these warnings in order to prevent recurrence; this ultimately led to the development of two major concepts in our system: 1) the three stages of activity-related musculoskeletal disorders, and 2) 'Tools to Fight Back®' (TTFB®). We were now ready to move into the primary prevention arena.

In 1985 we got our first opportunity to develop a primary prevention program; the challenge was to redesign a stretch break program that had proven ineffective. We developed a new program based on the theorem that all cumulative strain disorders are preventable if the individual recognizes warnings signals (i.e. stage 1), does something to control them during root issues (i.e. TTFB®), then uses the experience to establish new habits and behaviors to mitigate risks going forward.

The stretches we chose for the group program were also the primary

TTFB® we wanted the workers to use throughout the day, and at home (called micro-pauses) whenever warning signals developed. These became known as the 'opposite movements'. We provided training to perform the movements properly, plus why and how to use them – we made it clear that stretching as a group two times per day was not enough to prevent injuries. They needed micro-pauses and opposite movements and to connect these activities to better posture, body mechanics and exercise. We also had a contingency plan for 'outriggers' who didn't respond to the general information and tools and who required individualized attention. This became very important to managing this small group (10 – 20%) that is at high risk for chronic pain and disability.

Scrutinized closely by the company, they were pleasantly surprised to now have a program that not only worked but actually increased productivity. This was the beginning of a systematic and prevention-based approach for activity-related musculoskeletal disorders and disability. Our system is in a continuous state of evolution as we expand our service into new environments; integrating new information and knowledge, gaining new ideas, insights and skills from our colleagues, and most importantly from our patients and clients. This textbook provides the reader with a foundational body of information that is requisite to understanding our approach. Once you are familiar with this introductory material you are ready to learn our specific approach to regional musculoskeletal disorders and chronic musculoskeletal pain and disability. We recommend starting with the lower back.

Jean and I thank you for your interest in our approach and we hope that you find the information in this introductory book helpful to both you and your patients. This is to be followed by a series of books that identify our specific approach to the assessment, treatment and prevention of the following: 1) low back pain disorders and disability, 2) neck pain disorders and disability, 3) upper limb cumulative strain disorders, 4) lower limb degenerative and cumulative disorders, and 5) chronic musculoskeletal pain disorders and disability.

CONTENTS

	Acknowledgments	I
1	Introduction	8
2	Epidemiology of MSD	Pg 22
3	Research and Diagnostic Testing	Pg 32
4	Pain Definitions	Pg 44
5	History-taking	Pg 57
6	Basic Musculoskeletal Examination	Pg 74
7	Examination Conclusions	Pg 94
8	Manual Therapy Guidelines	Pg 103
9	Status Post Trauma	Pg 126
10	Cautions and Contraindications	Pg 142
11	Treatment Strategies	Pg 154
12	Long-term Management and Planning	Pg 168
	Abbreviations	Pg 179

ACKNOWLEDGMENTS

Thank you to our family for their love, support and putting up with our clinical practice obsession over the years. We are proud of you and the good citizens you have become, but not surprised that none of you went into healthcare as a profession. In addition we would like to thank the following important influences and colleagues:

James Cyriax for his logic, clinical discipline in patient selection and promoting the Physical Therapy profession as a first offensive weapon against musculoskeletal disorders.

Robin McKenzie for the many memories. His insights into assessment of activity-related back pain, the importance of patient self-management and the progression of force concepts were revolutionary. He paved the road for so many.

Mark Laslett, Paul Van Wijmen and Maynard Williams for all we shared and learned together in the early days of the Institute – you are our kindred spirits.

Brian Mulligan for taking manual therapy into the realm of patient movement, function and activity – you stimulated the most significant advancement in manual techniques in this generation. Your optimism, enthusiasm and pleasure when working with patients and students is contagious.

Gordon Waddell, Vert Mooney, Leonard Matheson and Nortin Hadler for their big picture and humble perspectives, commitment to evidence, and focus to keeping people active, able and empowered.

Lastly, to the thousands of patients and clients who have provided us with the experience needed to build and progress the system – you have kept us humble and focused, and taught us the most.

1 INTRODUCTION

MSDs are the most common clinical problem encountered in physical therapy practice; low back pain alone accounts for approximately 50% of all the patients who consume physical therapy treatment annually (Flynn 2011); neck/shoulder, wrist/hand and knee disorders are not far behind. The Duffy-Rath System© (DRS) is a prevention oriented approach to these common disorders, as defined by the World Health Organization (WHO): **primary prevention** – measures taken to prevent clinical manifestation; **secondary prevention** – measures taken to arrest development in the early stages; and **tertiary prevention** – measures taken to minimize consequences. Assessment and treatment of MSD is consequently a secondary or tertiary prevention activity unless the patient presents without signs or symptoms (i.e. in this case the care is primary prevention).

The World Health Organization (WHO) now recognizes a fourth prevention concern called; **quaternary prevention**. This is defined as methods to mitigate or avoid results of unnecessary or excessive interventions in the health system. This is a serious and growing problem in musculoskeletal healthcare (Deyo 2009; Pransky 2011). This is referred to as iatrogenesis in the literature and is defined as; the inadvertent adverse effect or complication resulting from treatment and/or advice of a healthcare practitioner(s). Regarding MSDs this includes any health-related disorder, disease, impairment or disability generated or exacerbated as a result of the treatment, advice and/or model utilized in providing care to the patient. We encourage and need all individual healthcare providers and their collective professions to understand this issue and actively facilitate practices that counter this concern – we must all step back and look at the big picture.

The Duffy-Rath System© strives to empower the patient. It is an assessment/reassessment driven process that attempts to build patient self-efficacy for the care of their own musculoskeletal health and function (i.e. musculoskeletal self-efficacy). Our approach to treatment and prevention of MSDs relies on the ability of the clinician to accurately identify the most relevant characteristics of the individual patient's problem and then effectively address the root causes. These characteristics are clinically expressed as symptoms, signs, interference with normal activities of daily living (ADL), and the patient's cognitive, psychological and emotional response to their problem.

The efficacy of our interventions is measured by the ability to eliminate or control these signs and symptoms and remove interference with the patient's normal ADL. This is how we challenge ourselves to prove the accuracy of our clinical and therapeutic conclusions, clinical models and therapeutic strategies. This challenge is accepted and measured one patient or client at a time. This requires basic skill and knowledge, discipline, and a focus to meeting the needs of each individual.

"Our mission is the prevention of musculoskeletal and lifestyle-related disorders and disability through education, training and research." Therefore our treatment strategies involve methods to actively involve the patient in their recovery. The intent is to recover faster and address root-cause issues that could lead to recurrence or to progression of the disorder. To summarize, the Duffy-Rath System© is an approach to the treatment and prevention of musculoskeletal disorders that is:

- Patient/client focused
- Response-based
- Activity/function oriented
- Outcome driven
- Striving for a long-term effect

The Duffy-Rath Treatment System© (DRS) is based on a BioPsychoSocial model. This is the most appropriate basis for managing disease, disorders and conditions that result from lifestyle factors and/or age-related and degenerative changes (Waddell 1987; Haldeman 1990; Bandura 1997). This does not mean we abandon the biomedical model; to the contrary, the biopsychosocial model expands it and provides an effective means of intervention when a clear diagnosis cannot be established or when treatments rendered based upon establishing a diagnosis are ineffective or only partially effective. This is particularly important when managing patients with chronic pain or activity-related disorders with non-mechanical presentations; and it is the operating model to address the long-term concerns for prevention of recurrence, progression and abnormal loss of activity tolerance.

Lastly, the DRS approach is especially sensitive to the importance of positive messaging. A clinician's conclusions and beliefs about the cause(s) and consequences of a MSD can have a significant and long-lasting impact on individuals – for the better or worse. Iatrogenic disability is a growing concern (Pransky 2011; Graves 2012). Our philosophy is to keep all patients as active as possible and appropriate through their recovery and to reinforce the importance of strategic activity as a therapeutic and preventative agent throughout life.

Axioms of the Duffy-Rath System©

1.   Healthcare goals for MSD – the ultimate measure of success in healthcare for MSDs is a reduced need for treatment combined with evidence that individuals are remaining active and able through a long and healthy life. This indicates that primary and secondary prevention efforts are working. A literal definition of healthcare insinuates preventative actions and measures, whereas treatment is actually illness care with the intent of restoring the individual back to health (Rath 2002).

When treatment is required, success is measured by effectiveness (i.e. elimination/control of relevant signs and symptoms, and a safe return to normal levels of activity) and efficiency (i.e. the time, effort and costs) – but since many MSDs resolve spontaneously, results of treatment need to be compared to natural history and more importantly to the long-term effect of the intervention; i.e. preventing recurrence, progression and preserving the ability of the patient to remain active.

Most MSDs are <u>not</u> a product of an accident or frank trauma, rather they are a result of biomechanical and activity-related (lifestyle) habits, the physical environments of daily life, and the influence of a variety of psychosocial variables. Therefore we need to help the patient build self-management skills to address root issues for both short and long-term efficacy.

2. Five Core Elements (CE) to the DRS – each of these five domains need to be addressed to restore, maintain or enhance physical function related to the musculoskeletal system. The combined effect of all five elements is key, relying on one or a couple is not adequate.

CE 1 Biomechanical control – habits that promote the conservation of mechanical stress and strain on the connective tissues of the musculoskeletal system through improved posture (i.e. axial alignment) and body mechanics (i.e. control of center of mass within base of support, and using leverage to an advantage). This is foundational to a musculoskeletal prevention approach.

CE 2 Effective use of Tools to Fight Back® (TTFB®) – routine behaviors and actions that invest in cumulative wellness to prevent cumulative, degenerative disorders and sustain safe physical performance capabilities. This involves development of a personalized system of tools that balances stress and strain patterns of physical demand, effectively controls warning signals, and promotes habits that service and maintain the other core elements.

The process of developing a personalized TTFB® system involves a sequence of actions in response to warning signals: 1) correct posture, 2) correct body mechanics/ergonomics, 3) take a micro-pause (i.e. made strategic by using the 'opposite movement rule') and 4) perform the specific procedure identified to control the symptoms or signs. Control of warning signals establishes a 'cause and effect' and repetition leads to habit change. This experience is then connected to the other core elements.

CE 3 Healthy (adequate) ROM – a healthy joint is able to move to and from a mid-range (neutral) position to an end range position without pain (end range is the point where slack is removed from the joint capsule and supportive ligaments). A healthy joint also has a normal mechanical and symptom response when overpressure is applied at end range (i.e. a sensation of stretch / strain that increases proportionally as the overpressure is increased). And lastly, there are no adverse consequence when the joint is returned to mid-range (i.e. the capsule and ligaments have maintained normal elasticity and integrity and there is no lasting symptom response). This response would be found in all directions that the joint complex is designed to move when healthy.

In addition to joint motion, the soft tissues must have adequate extensibility to allow biomechanical control relative to the individual's normal physical demands (home, work and play). This is especially important for the muscles that cross more than one joint (e.g. hamstrings, hip flexors etc.) and the nerve tunnels connecting the spine to the limbs.

Note: obviously some patients are unable to restore a normal end range response to overpressure (e.g. a relevant spinal instability, joint trauma, connective tissue abnormality etc.). In this case maintaining as large a symptom-free mid-range as possible is the goal, and improving soft-tissue extensibility to maintain the best biomechanical control is the motion target.

CE 4 Strategic strength & conditioning – there needs to be adequate power, endurance and motor control to maintain biomechanical control under progressively greater physical loads (i.e. when lifting, carrying, pushing, pulling, reaching, throwing, etc.). Additionally, there needs to be a cushion between the individual's physical ability (i.e. exercise tolerance and maximal safe exertion capacity) and the physical demands of their lifestyle for the prevention of fatigue-related MSD. Demand levels vary tremendously so the approach needs to be specific to the individual.

CE 5 Musculoskeletal Self-efficacy – belief and confidence in the ability to control musculoskeletal health and physical performance capabilities is essential. This is especially important in the face of developing problems or frank injury, and in the long-term requires the integration of habits and routines that reinforce the previous elements. The knowledge and skills gained by reacting constructively to warning signals, symptoms or signs reinforces the continuance of activity and ability.

3.   **The Three Stages of Musculoskeletal Disorders** – cumulative strain disorders (CSD) are the product of mechanical and physiological demands that in a single dose are not capable of doing harm or damage to connective tissues. Damage may eventually result when repeated or sustained biomechanical and physiological demands are too frequent and/or sustained for too long, interfering with the ability of the tissues to recover and eventually leading to structural failure. This is a description of fatigue failure.

The only way the body has to communicate fatigue is through symptoms and we call these symptoms 'warning signals'. Symptoms of fatigue are a normal response and will fully resolve without consequence unless the pattern of fatigue is allowed to accumulate; then the fatigue response grows and may eventually become abnormal. The three stages concept is designed to help the individual recognize the distinction between normal and abnormal fatigue-related responses in a way that promotes musculoskeletal self-efficacy.

Stage one – this is the 'warning signal' stage where the symptoms produced are the product of mechanical fatigue in the supportive joint structures and/or physiological fatigue in the neuromuscular system. Once the load that produced the fatigue is removed (i.e. change position, stop the activity etc.) the symptoms quickly or immediately subside, there are no relevant (symptom producing) signs, nor any interference with the individual's normal function and activity levels. The symptoms are transient and there are no physical signs directly relevant to the pain. All cumulative MSDs pass through this stage, so by definition they are all preventable because in this stage there is no relevant diagnosis or disorder.

Stage two – stage 1 progresses because the fatigue-related exposures are not interrupted enough to allow recovery and the source activity has not been adequately or effectively managed. The symptoms progress by persisting after the load is removed, expanding in location or intensity, and starting to have consequences to function and activity-tolerance. In addition, signs that are relevant to the symptom production emerge.

Initially the symptoms and signs are not specific enough to identify structural damage or a specific pathological diagnosis with accuracy; hence this is called the 'nonspecific stage'. This represents 70 – 90 percent of all activity-related spine pain patients and is a progression from stage one or the result of a minor trauma (i.e. sprain, strain, 'back or neck out' etc.). In the extremities this represents a minor disorder regardless of whether or not the structural source can be accurately identified. Most stage 2 disorders are rapidly reversible with early intervention (secondary prevention) provided the approach addresses root issues or simply because of a favorable natural history.

Stage 2 disorders can progress towards stage 3, or simply fail to resolve for a variety of reasons. When a nonspecific problem becomes chronic and/or leads to disability recovery is slower and more difficult.

Stage three – stage 3 results when the plan of care during stage 2 is unable to effectively control root issues, or it is the result of trauma, or it is the nature of the particular problem. In any regard the symptoms and signs have worsened and are now consistent with specific, more significant pathology. There is now unequivocal and well correlated physical examination and diagnostic evidence. Common diagnoses include; acute disc herniation with radiculopathy, a ruptured rotator cuff, spinal stenosis, ACL tear, etc.

Many of these disorders are reversible, even without surgery but they are slower to respond to treatment and some never restore a normal examination. Most of those with normal or average lifestyle demands recover their activity-tolerance, but some with vigorous demands may require permanent change or modifications. This is the only group where surgery should be considered, but candidates need to be selected carefully. A long-term focus is critical, but can be difficult because of the inability to effect rapid change. This sometimes leads to hasty, short-term oriented decisions that are ultimately not productive.

4. **Tools To Fight Back® System** – this is the DRS nickname; TTFB® for short. TTFBs are changes in posture, body mechanics and work set-up; as well as opposite movements or self-applied procedures that interrupt the accumulation of stress and strain and help control relevant symptoms, signs and/or problems with physical function. When symptoms or signs appear the TTFB® must reduce or eliminate them; i.e. it is only a TTFB® if it is effective.

Discovering these tools provides the 'cause and effect' experience that is critical to a successful outcome and facilitating musculoskeletal self-efficacy. The search is an enjoyable and rewarding aspect of clinical practice.

5. **Organization of Interventions** – the DRS strives for both effectiveness and efficiency of musculoskeletal healthcare with a positive, long-term effect. Interactive patient education and training links treatment and prevention, providing a foundation for building musculoskeletal self-efficacy. The following organization of intervention requirements and expectations is consistent with the prevention continuum. Our hope is for conservative, physical therapy based interventions to shift to level one and two.

- **Level 1 (education & training)** – patients or clients in stage one or early stage two do not require more than education and training to resolve their problem. The critical issue is to provide them with tools that help them effectively self-manage and prevent warning signals from progressing. Once an effective TTFB® system is established they should be provided with long-term instructions to address the five core elements.
- **Level 2 (simple physical therapy)** – stage two disorders with mechanically-responsive signs and symptoms are fun to treat

because they are (invariably) rapidly reversible using a classic mechanical approach; e.g. McKenzie, Mulligan, Cyriax etc. These patients can gain full control over their problem quickly. The long-term is addressed as in level 1, but with special consideration to the nature of their specific MSD and the TTFB® system that resolved their mechanical disorder.

- **Level 3 (complex physical therapy)** – these are stage two or three patients that cannot gain rapid control over their symptoms and signs and/or restore normal tolerance to full activity quickly. They require a remodeling approach to regain full or potential control. This includes the need to implement a gradual, but progressive stretching or strength and conditioning program targeted to specific functional goals. The TTFB® system for this group improves throughout the course of recovery and segues to level-one training for a positive long-term impact.

- **Level 4 (rehabilitation)** – these are stage two or three patients that have developed a chronic pain disability and are now out of work. They require a multidisciplinary team approach, or at least a coordination of the various disciplines involved, all working towards the common goal of returning the patient to activity. The TTFB® concept remains important, but has to be altered when the signs and symptoms do not exhibit mechanical behavior.

6.   **Musculoskeletal self-efficacy** – we have used this term repeatedly so let's describe it further. We coined this term in the 1990s to focus attention to the importance of an individual's belief and confidence in their ability to prevent and manage MSD and their physical performance capabilities. There is a substantial body of evidence for the importance of self-efficacy in healthcare, particularly with lifestyle-related and degenerative disorders (Bandura 1997). There is further evidence of the importance of self-efficacy in physical performance, return to function and overcoming chronic pain disability (Jensen 1991; Kaivanto 1995; Lackner 1996; 1999). A resilient self-belief system is also important to quaternary prevention.

In the next chapter evidence-based risk factors related to activity-related musculoskeletal disorders (ARMSD) are reviewed. Many of the identified risks for the onset of ARMSD are associated with postures, biomechanics, physical work demands, etc. However, most of the factors associated with resulting disability are psychosocial; fear avoidance beliefs, depression, poor coping skills, a lack of self-efficacy etc. So, a key question is, "how can we facilitate positive change in these beliefs and behaviors"; is it possible?

There is evidence that we can, but it is found mainly in the behavioral sciences (Jensen 1991; Kaivanto 1995). Bandura has been a champion in this field of study, and his description of self-efficacy is applicable to the prevention of ARMSD; i.e. self-efficacy is a "resilient self-belief system in the face of obstacles" (Bandura 1989; Nicholas 2007). A new field of research has emerged relevant to this; "Self-Determination Theory" (Deci EL, Ryan RM 2002). This has significant applicability and it is nice to see the recognition of self-efficacy emerging in the physical therapy research literature (Harrison 2004).

In the DRS we attempt to facilitate the patient's musculoskeletal self-efficacy by several means; 1) first by accurately isolating their relevant signs and symptoms (RSSx), 2) second, by providing them with TTFB® to control the RSSx when present (i.e. cause and effect), 3) third, by providing a simple explanation and rationale they can apply to control the problem, and 4) by remaining positive, supportive and encouraging until they integrate the information and skills. This is consistent with evidence of methods to improve patient autonomy in self-determination theory research (Williams 2002).

In addition to belief and behavior, habits have a significant impact on the success or failure in preventing ARMSD and sustaining physical performance capability while aging. Recent research evidence suggests the importance of repetition, connection to goal setting and providing an environment for positive change in habitual behaviors (Muraven 1999; Wood 2005; 2007; Neal 2006; Baumeister 2007). Once we identify the most effective postural TTFB® we stress the importance of repetition until the biomechanical behavior is integrated into the sensory-motor system and now automatic; i.e. a change in habit. The flow diagram below indicates how we attempt to help the patient or client adopt good biomechanical habits and behavior, and how we facilitate musculoskeletal self-efficacy.

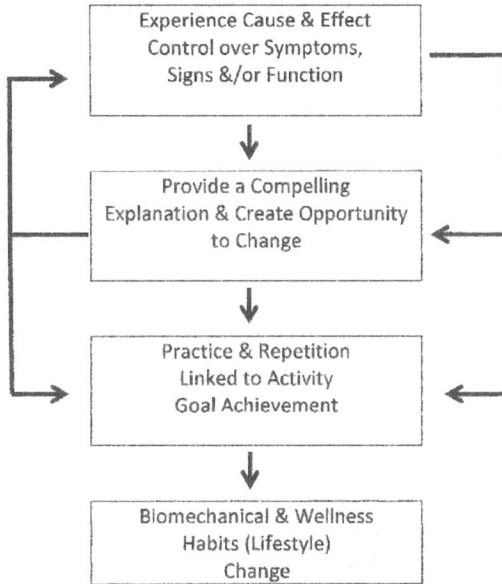

```
        ┌─────────────────────────────┐
        │   Experience Cause & Effect │
    ──→ │   Control over Symptoms,    │ ──┐
        │   Signs &/or Function       │   │
        └─────────────────────────────┘   │
                     ↓                     │
        ┌─────────────────────────────┐   │
        │     Provide a Compelling     │   │
    ┌── │ Explanation & Create Opportunity │ ←─┘
        │        to Change             │
        └─────────────────────────────┘
                     ↓
        ┌─────────────────────────────┐
        │   Practice & Repetition      │
    ──→ │    Linked to Activity        │ ←──
        │     Goal Achievement         │
        └─────────────────────────────┘
                     ↓
        ┌─────────────────────────────┐
        │   Biomechanical & Wellness  │
        │     Habits (Lifestyle)       │
        │         Change               │
        └─────────────────────────────┘
```

We refer to the results of systematic reviews and meta-analyses throughout the book. In order to evaluate the quality and strength of the evidence presented, clinicians should be familiar with the PRISMA Statement (Preferred Reporting Items for Systematic reviews and Meta-Analysis) for transparent reporting of systematic reviews and meta-analyses (Moher 2009; 2010). In 2001 Altman et. al. published the revised CONSORT (consolidated standards of reporting trials) statement as part of a continued attempt to improve the quality of research reporting in the medical literature. It is important to rank the relative strength of evidence according to these types of standards when developing assessment and treatment approaches; we call this the 'external evidence-basis' for clinical practice and this represents the current trend in healthcare science.

Our position has always been that **internal evidence trumps external evidence** when it comes to managing patients. Internal evidence is the observed, measured and actual response of the individual patient to the care provided. Many times what works in the clinic does not have external evidence support; at least not yet. Clinical practice is the incubator for new ideas, strategies, procedures and techniques – the external evidence eventually catches-up by sorting out what is reproducible and holds generalizable truth. As a patient advocate you need to listen carefully, identify the most relevant findings and factors for each individual, and do whatever is required to optimize the benefits of their treatment. Clinical practice is a consecutive series of single-case studies designed to find what achieves the best result with each and every patient.

References Chapter 1:

Abenhaim L, Rossignol M, Gobeille D, Bonvalot Y, Fines P, Scott S: The prognostic consequences in the making of the initial medical diagnosis of work-related back injuries. Spine 20 (7): 791-795, 1995.

Altman DG, Schulz KF, Moher D, et al. The revised CONSORT statement for reporting randomized trials: explanation and elaboration. Ann Intern Med 134:663–94, 2001.

Bandura A. Perceived self-efficacy in the exercise of personal agency. The Psychologist: Bul Brit Psychol Soc 10: 411-24, 1989.

Bandura, A. Self-efficacy: The exercise of control. WH Freeman and Co., New York, 1997.
Deci EL, Ryan RM, Editors. Handbook of Self-Determination Research. University of Rochester Press, Rochester, NY, 2002.

Baumeister RF, Vohs KD, Tice DM. The strength model of self-control. Curr Directions in Psych Sci 16 (6): 351-55, 2007.

Deyo RA, Mirza SK, Turner JA, Martin BI. Overtreating chronic back pain: time to back off? JABFM 22 (1): 62 – 68, 2009.

Flynn TW, Smith B, Chou R. Appropriate use of diagnostic imaging in low back pain: a reminder that unnecessary imaging may do as much harm as good. JOSPT 41 (11): 838-46, 2011.

Graves JM, Fulton-Kehoe D, Jarvik JG, Franklin GM. Early imaging for acute low back pain: one-year health and disability outcomes among Washington Stare workers. Spine 37 (18): 1617-27, 2012.

Haldeman S: Presidential Address, NASS: failure of the pathology model to predict back pain. Spine 15(7): 718-724, 1990.

Harrison AL. The influence of pathology, pain, balance, and self-efficacy on function in women with osteoarthritis of the knee. Phys Ther 84 (9): 822-31, 2004.

Jensen MP, Turner JA, Romano JM. Self-efficacy and outcome expectancy relationship to chronic pain, coping strategies and adjustment. Pain 44 (3):263–9, 1991.

Kaivanto KK, Estlander AM, Moneta GB, Vanharanta H. Isokinetic performance in low back pain patients: the predictive power of the self-efficacy scale. J Occup Rehab 5 (2): 87 – 99, 1995.

Lackner JM, Carosella AM, Feuerstein M. Pain expectancies, pain, and functional self-efficacy expectancies as determinants of disability in patients with chronic low back disorders. J Consult Clin Psychol 1996;64:212–20.

Lackner JM, Carosella AM, The Relative Influence of Perceived Pain Control, Anxiety, and Functional Self Efficacy on Spinal Function Among Patients With Chronic Low Back Pain Spine 24 (21): 2254–2261, 1999.

Moher D, Liberati A, Tetzlaff J, Altman DG, The PRISMA Group (2009). Preferred Reporting Items for Systematic Reviews and Meta-Analyses: The PRISMA Statement. BMJ 2009; 339: b2535, doi: 10.1136/bmj.b2535.

Moher D, Liberati A, Tetzlaff J, Altman DG, The PRISMA Group. Preferred Reporting Items for Systematic Reviews and Meta-Analyses: The PRISMA Statement. Int J Surg 2010; doi:10.1016/ j.ijsu.2010.02.007

Muraven M, Baumeister RF, Tice DM. Longitudinal improvement of self-regulation through practice: building self-control strength through repeated exercise. J Social Pyschology 139 (4): 446-57, 1999.

Neal DT, Wood W, Quinn JM. Habits-a repeat performance. Curr Dir Psychol Sci 15 (4): 198-202, 2006.

Nicholas MK. The pain self-efficacy questionnaire: taking pain into account. Europ J Pain 11: 153-63, 2007.

Pransky G, Borkan JM, Young AE, Cherkin DC. Are we making progress? The tenth international forum for primary care research on low back pain. Spine 36 (19): 1608-14, 2011.

Rath W. Spinal manipulation and the prevention of dysfunction and disability. Combined Sections APTA, Orthopaedic Section: The Integration of Manual Therapy & Musculoskeletal Wellness, Boston, Feb. 23, 2002.

Waddell G: A new clinical model for the treatment of low-back pain: biopsychosocial. Spine 12 (7): 632-644, 1987.

Williams GC. Improving patient's health through supporting the autonomy of patients and providers. IN; Deci EL, Ryan RM, Editors. <u>Handbook of Self-Determination Research</u>. University of Rochester Press, Rochester, NY, 2002; pp. 233 – 254.

Wood W, Neal DT. A new look at habits and the habit-goal interface. Psych Rev 114 (4): 843 – 63, 2007.

Wood W, Witt MG, Tam L. Changing circumstances, disrupting habits. J Personality and Social Psychology 88 (6): 918 – 33, 2005.

2 EPIDEMIOLOGY
MUSCULOSKELETAL DISORDERS & DISABILITY

Epidemiology involves the study of incidence and prevalence of disease and disorders; including investigations of source, cause, and/or predisposing factors. Having basic knowledge of the epidemiology of MSDs and disability is critical to clinical practice and healthcare research. The STROBE Statement (**ST**rengthening the **R**eporting of **OB**servational studies in **E**pidemiology) is a resource to help clinicians evaluate the quality and strength of epidemiologic trials (Vanderbroucke 2007).

Musculoskeletal clinicians need a solid understanding of epidemiology relevant to each MSD target. This includes a working knowledge of the incidence, prevalence, natural history, risk factors for onset and/or recurrence, risk factors for reporting to a medical or healthcare practitioner, and risk factors associated with development of chronic pain and disability. Ultimately the public needs this information to make better, well-informed decisions.

Prevalence of MSD in the general population

Looking at the prevalence of regional musculoskeletal pain in the general population (i.e. regardless of occupation or employment status) is a good starting point. Prevalence is the frequency of a disease or disorder in the population – identified by the timeframe of the study (e.g. point prevalence, 1-month, 3-month, 1-year, etc.) and case definitions for the target MSD. This should not be confused with incidence which identifies the rate of occurrence of new cases for a disease or disorder.

Table 2-1 provides the 1-month and 3-month prevalence of regional musculoskeletal pain in adults (≥ 18 years) in the United States in 2010; the results range from 7.1% for hip pain to 29.1% for low back pain (National Center for Health Statistics 2011). Back, knee, neck and shoulder pain top the list – severe headache is also quite prevalent, however the source of many severe headaches is not musculoskeletal.

Table 2-1 There is a high prevalence of MSD in the general US population according to a 2010 survey; in addition approximately 1/3 of those surveyed (≥ 18 years of age) reported having joint pain and significant activity restriction in the past month (National Center for Health Statistics. Health, United States, 2010: tables 52, 53).

Severe Headache	LBP	Neck Pain	Shoulder Pain	Finger Pain	Hip Pain	Knee Pain	Any Joint Pain
16.1% 3-month	29.1% 3-month	15.1% 3-month	9.0% 1-month	7.6% 1-month	7.1% 1-month	19.5 1-month	32.0% 1-month

Missing from the table above is information about prevalence of wrist/hand symptoms; a common musculoskeletal complaint seen in clinical practice. Atroshi et. al. (1999) reported a point prevalence of 14.4% for carpal tunnel symptoms (95% CI: 13-15.8%); the conclusion of the study was that carpal tunnel like symptoms are common in the general population – approximately one in five adults. However the study had a follow-up physical and electrophysiological examination for those who reported symptoms and compared this with a control group of individuals without symptoms. There was a higher rate of abnormal electrophysiological testing in the control (asymptomatic) group – this confounding factor of false positive diagnostic testing is addressed throughout this book and the DRS in general. for it has a profound impact on MSD treatment and prevention, iatrogenesis and self-efficacy.

Risk Factors for MSD

The identification of risk factors for the onset of MSD is obviously important for primary and secondary prevention; strategies need to prioritize control of the greatest risks. The literature has many trials focused on investigating for work-related risk factors. This is understandable considering the significant socioeconomic impact of work-related MSD (WRMSD); e.g. 85.9 billion dollars spent for US healthcare costs associated with low back and neck pain alone in 2005 (Martin 2008). However, people are exposed to many of the same risk factors at home, with recreational activities, and during their commute to and from work. Isolating the role of work factors alone is actually quite difficult.

Da Costa et. al. (2010) conducted a well-designed systematic review of the literature reporting risks for WRMSD. The review was limited to studies of acceptable design and the strength of the evidence was given a 3-point rating; strong evidence, reasonable evidence or insufficient evidence. Table 2-2 lists the results of the review for 7 musculoskeletal regions; it should be noted that none of the factors listed had strong evidence – further evidence that risk is multifactorial.

Table 2-2: Da Costa et. al. 2010 published the results of a systematic review of case-control and cohort studies of risk factors for WRMSD; the following are the risk factors with reasonable evidence for causality – there were no factors identified to have 'strong evidence' for a causal relationship. 1,990 references reviewed; accepted were 22 studies of the upper limb, 12 of the lower back, 7 of the neck and 6 for the lower limb. There were also 5 nonspecific studies and 2 related to fibromyalgia not included in the table.

Neck	Shoulder	Wrist/hand	Low Back	Hip	Knee	Foot/ankle
Psychosocial Smoking, Female Awkward posture Co-morbidities	Heavy work Psychosocial (limited investigation)	Computer work, Heavy work, Awkward posture, Repetitive work, High BMI, Older age, Female	Heavy work, Awkward posture Lifting, Psychosocial High BMI, Younger age	Heavy work Lifting (limited investigation)	Awkward posture, Lifting Repetition Co-morbidities	Needs further research

As a general rule, the risk for the onset of musculoskeletal pain can be attributed to physical demand factors; i.e. highly repetitive and/or forceful tasks, continuous reaching and manual manipulation, prolonged static loading and awkward or extreme postures etc. (NIOSH 1997; Humphreys 1998; Vingard 2000). However the strongest factors associated with likelihood of a worker reporting LBP was having previously reported one, work dissatisfaction and a poor relationship with supervisor or co-workers (Bigos 1995). Next we will look at risk factors for chronic musculoskeletal pain and disability; ultimately a prevention oriented approach needs to identify and address all the factors (bio-psycho-social) as they apply to the individual patient.

Risk Factors for MSD Disability and Chronic Musculoskeletal Pain

Turner et. al. (2008) identified the following baseline predictors of work disability with back injuries: severe functional disability ratings (Roland Morris Disability Questionnaire; RDQ), the number of pain sites, description of job as 'hectic', no light duty accommodation, previous injury with extended sick leave and specialty of first health care provider (i.e. chiropractic fared best in this study). "This confirms clinical impressions that patients with similar examination and imaging findings vary in pain and disability outcomes, likely because of factors other than biologic ones."

Margarita Nordin (2001), the first physical therapist and female president of the International Society for the Study of the Lumbar Spine (ISSLS) provides an excellent overview of evidence-based risk factors associated with reporting LBP and those associated with LBP disability in an occupational setting. Her message stresses the importance of keeping work-related LBP patients active, and getting them back to work as soon as possible as a component of their therapy and rehabilitation; table 3 lists an overview of these evidence-based factors. The DRS philosophy has always been; "keep them working while recovering – don't put them out in the first place".

Table 2-3: Nordin 2001 identified evidence-based factors associated with reporting a LBP problem and those associated with LBP disability in an occupational setting; she also identified factors associated with delaying the recovery from the onset of a work-related LBP problem.

Reporting LBP		LBP Disability		Delaying Recovery
Smoking Lack of job support Job dissatisfaction Work exposure to whole body vibration Lifting	Company down-sizing Unemployment Lack of social support at work Age Previous back pain history	Gender Abnormal gait Work exposure to whole body vibration Co-morbidity	Age Previous back pain Specific diagnosis Perception of disability Type of intervention	Maintain the old belief that long-term rest is healthy Medicalization of a condition with no objective clinical findings Give long-term passive treatment Don't communicate with the workplace

In general, the major risk factors associated with chronic musculoskeletal pain and disability are psychosocial – Table 2-4 summarizes these findings in a cross-section of studies. Risk factors include passive coping, catastrophizing, fear-avoidance behaviors, depression, anxiety, lack of control over the work environment and a moderate association to a blue collar occupation (Linton 2000; Ijzelenberg 2005; Bergström 2007; Carroll 2008). The "New Zealand acute low back pain guide" (ACC 1997) is a good resource to review these "yellow flags"; i.e. psychosocial and other factors that can interfere with a patient's recovery from LBP and contribute to chronic pain disability. These same factors apply to WRMSD in general.

Table 2-4: A selection of studies and systematic reviews looking at risk factors for chronic musculoskeletal pain and disability indicate that psychosocial issues predominate and need to be identified and addressed in treatment and prevention strategies.

Study	Design	Population	Risk Factors
Armenian et. al. 1998	Population-based Cohort	1,920 patients 1,715 control	Major depression was a significant risk factor for chronic physical illness and disability.
Picavet et. al. 2002	Population-based Cohort	1,571	Follow-up found kinesiophobia to predict LBP and disability even when there were no symptoms/problems at original survey.
Pincus et. al. 2002	Sys review	25 publications (18 cohorts)	Distress, depressive mood and somatization are predictors. Need to address coping strategies and fear avoidance to prevent disability.
Denison et. al. 2004	Component of Prospective Cohort	Two samples: n1 = 210 n2 = 161	Self-efficacy and fear avoidance more predictive of disability than pain intensity and pain duration.
IJzelenberg et. al. 2005	Longitudinal with 6-mo follow-up	505 workers 407 (81%) at follow-up	Older age and living alone predictive for LBP disability. Living alone and female predictive of neck/upper extremity disability.
Sivertsen et. al. 2006	Population-based Cohort	92,100	Insomnia is a strong predictor of disability; independent of socio-demographic and shift-work status.
Mallen et. al. 2007	Systematic review (Observational cohort in primary care)	45 studies identified for review	11 factors found to be associated with poor outcome with musculoskeletal pain: higher pain severity, longer pain duration, multiple-site pain, previous pain episodes, anxiety and/or depression, higher somatic perceptions and/or distress, adverse coping strategies, low social support, older age, higher baseline disability and greater movement restriction.
Ropponen et. al. 2011a	Twin Cohort Study	24,043 over 30 years	Risk for disability due to MSD/OA predicted by comorbidities, educational level and social class.
Ropponen et. al. 2011b	Population-based	1,387,166 men born bet 1951 - 1976	Hand grip/body weight ratio is strongly and inversely associated with pension disability due to MSD later in life.
Gjesdal et. al 2011	Prospective Cohort (Norway)	37,942 woman 26,307 men > 8 weeks sick leave	Woman at greater risk for disability than men. Socioeconomic status (lower income) increased risk. Diagnosis of myalgia/ fibromyalgia > OA had poorer prognosis. Back pain and non-traumatic UE disorders = 50% of cases.

After looking at the evidence for prevalence in the general population, risk for onset, report and chronic pain/disability, it becomes apparent how difficult it is to isolate work factors as the cause of MSD. Although well intended, workers' compensation systems and OSHA often place too much blame and responsibility on the employer and not enough on the individual. When it comes to prevention of activity related musculoskeletal disorders (ARMSD) and disability you have to address the relevant factors – hence the need for a biopsychosocial approach. This is evidenced in emerging research that has found a strong association between stress factors in an individual's life, entitled "work-life conflict" (WLC), and a five-fold higher prevalence rate and a six-fold increased relative risk for MSD (Hämmig et. al. 2011). The interplay of relevant factors at work, home and play all need to be addressed.

Natural History of MSD

The natural history of any disease or disorder is the expected timeframe and course of recovery when no treatment or intervention is provided. Knowledge of this is imperative to managing patients effectively, yet surprisingly little information is known about the natural history for many MSDs. Healthcare is supposed to be guided by the rule; "first do no harm" – without knowing the natural history how can you tell whether any harm has been done?

In general we can presume that the natural history for most MSD is quite favorable; most do resolve with a "tincture of time". Unless diseased, our biology is resilient and designed to survive – when injured we heal. Undoubtedly some MSDs fail to spontaneously resolve as evidenced by the growing number of people disabled with chronic musculoskeletal pain; recovery involves more than biological repair and remodeling.

Nonetheless it is a minority of patients with MSD that become chronic and disabled (roughly 20% ±). This is the group that suffers most, have the greatest consequences and represent the majority of costs related to MSD. Preventing chronic pain and disability should be the primary target – this requires a biopsychosocial model of action.

The natural history for back and neck pain problems has been researched and explored more than any other MSD. The Quebec Task

Force report (Spitzer 1987) defined chronic as an activity-related spinal disorder (ARSD) that persisted greater than seven weeks simply because 90% of the cases should have recovered within that timeframe. Failure to recover implies undetected or inadequately addressed factors; diagnosis and treatment should be completely reassessed when patients have not resolved their back or neck pain within 2 months.

The bottom-line for natural history is there are two prevailing and applicable constructs: 1) one which says that most cases respond favorably with or without treatment, and 2) another which states that many cases never fully recover, experiencing varying periods and degrees of remission and exacerbation (Croft 1998). This later construct is epitomized in the Neck Pain Task Force Report in 2008; "Neck pain is viewed as an episodic occurrence over a lifetime with variable recovery between episodes" (Guzman et. al. 2008).

These two constructs appear diametrically opposed. The common factor is the fact that in either case recurrence is a significant issue. A recurrent episode is defined by a period of full recovery in between; this group exhibits a favorable natural history, but with each recurrence the chance of pathological progression or chronic pain and disability increases. A recurrent flare-up never had a time period of full recovery; the condition is chronic and this group is the opposite example. This group requires an approach that minimizes, or when possible eliminates the consequences of the chronic disorder. In both cases patient treatment needs a long-term focus; this is one of the underlying principles in the DRS – promoting musculoskeletal self-efficacy.

A last consideration for reviewing the literature about natural history of MSD is to carefully inspect the study population. Many studies take place after the individual has sought treatment, yet this may represent only a small percentage of people that experience the problem; e.g. only about 10 – 15% of people that experience back pain seek treatment. You cannot be labeled to have chronic pain nor deemed disabled if you never go to a doctor; so there is inherent bias with those who become patients. And, there is growing evidence that iatrogenic disability is a growing concern (Abenhaim 1995; Nordin 2001; Pransky 2011). And, as previously mentioned, if the study population is limited to workers; other lifestyle factors that could influence onset and failure to recover are overlooked.

References Chapter 2

Abenhaim L, Rossignol M, Gobeille D, Bonvalot Y, Fines P, Scott S: The prognostic consequences in the making of the initial medical diagnosis of work-related back injuries. Spine 20 (7): 791-795, 1995.

ACC and the National Health Committee (1997). New Zealand acute low back pain guide. Ministry of Health & Accident Rehabilitation and Compensation Insurance Corporation. Wellington, New Zealand

Atroshi I, Gummesson C, Johnsson R, Ornstein E, Ranstam J and Rosen I Prevalence of carpal tunnel syndrome in a general population. JAMA 281(2):153-158, 1999.

Armenian HK, Pratt LA, Gallo J, Eaton WW. Psychopathology as a predictor of disability: a population-based follow-up study in Baltimore, Maryland. Am J Epidem 148 (3): 269 – 75, 1998.

Bergström G, Bodin L, Bertilsson H, Jensen B. Risk factors for new episodes of sick leave due to neck or back pain in working population: a prospective study with an 18-month and a three-year follow-up. Occup Environ Med 64 (4): 279-87, 2007.

Bigos S, Battie M, Spengler D, et. al. A prospective study of work perceptions and psychosocial factors affecting the report of back injury. Spine 1991: 16 (6) 1-6.

Carroll LJ, Hogg-Johnson S, van der Velde G, et, al. Course and Prognostic Factors for Neck Pain in the General Population: Results of the Bone and Joint Decade 2000-2010 Task Force on Neck Pain and Its Associated Disorders Spine 33(4S) : S75-82, 2008.

Croft PR, Macfarlane GJ, Papageogiou AC, Thomas E, Silman AJ. Outcome of low back pain in general practice: a prospective study. MNJ 316: 1356-59, 1998.

Da Costa BR, Vieira ER. Risk factors for work-related musculoskeletal disorders: a systematic review of recent longitudinal studies. Am J Ind Med 53 (3): 285-323, 2010.

Denison E, Asenlöf P, Lindberg P. Self-efficacy, fear avoidance, and pain intensity as predictors of disability in subacute and chronic musculoskeletal pain patients in primary health care. Pain 111(3): 245-52, 2004.

Gjesdal S, Bratberg E, Maeland JG. Gender differences in disability after sickness absence with musculoskeletal disorders: five-year prospective study of 37,942 women and 2,307 men. BMC Musculoskeletal Disord. 2011 Feb 7; 12:37.

Introduction to the Duffy-Rath System©

Guzman J, Hurwitz EL, Carroll LJ, Haldeman S, Côté P, Carragee EJ, Peloso PM, van der Velde G, Holm LW, Hogg-Johnson S, Nordin M, Cassidy JD. A New Conceptual Model of Neck Pain: Linking Onset, Course, and Care: The Bone and Joint Decade 2000-2010 Task Force on Neck Pain and Its Associated Disorders Spine 33(4S): S14-23, 2008.

Hämmig O, Knecht M, Läubli T, Bauer GF. Work-life conflict and musculoskeletal disorders: a cross-sectional study of an unexplored association. BMC Musculoskelet Disord 2011 Mar 16;12:60.

Hult L. Cervical, dorsal and lumbar spinal syndromes: a field investigation of a non-selected material of 1200 workers in different occupations with special reference to disc degeneration and so-called muscular rheumatism. ACTA Orth Scand 17 [Suppl]: 1-197, 1954.

Humphreys SC, Hodges SD, Patwardhan A, Eck JC, Covington LA, Sartori M. The Natural History of the Cervical Foramen in Symptomatic and Asymptomatic Individuals Aged 20-60 Years as Measured by Magnetic Resonance Imaging: A Descriptive Approach Spine. 23(20): 2180-2184, 1998.

IJzelenberg W, Burdorf A. Risk Factors for Musculoskeletal Symptoms and Ensuing Health Care Use and Sick Leave. Spine 30 (13): 1550–56, 2005.

Linton SJ, Andersson T. Can Chronic Disability Be Prevented?: A Randomized Trial of a Cognitive-Behavior Intervention and Two Forms of Information for Patients With Spinal Pain. Spine. 25(21):2825-2831, 2000.

Luime JJ, Koes BW, Hendriksen IJM, Verhagen AP, Miedema HS, Verhaar JAN. Prevalence and incidence of shoulder pain in the general population: a systematic review. Scand J Rheum 33 (2): 73-81, 2004.

Mallen CD, Peat G, Thomas E, Dunn KM, Croft PR. Prognostic factors for musculoskeletal pain in primary care: a systematic review. Br J Gen Practice 57 (541): 655-661, 2007.

Martin BI, Deyo RA, Mirza SK, et. al. Expenditures and health status among adults with back and neck problems. JAMA 2008; 299:656-664, http://dx.doi.org/10.1001/jama.299.6.656.

National Center for Health Statistics. Health, United States, 2010: With Special Feature on Death and Dying. Hyattsville, MD. 2011 (http://www.cdc.gov/nchs/data/hus/hus10.pdf)

NIOSH. Musculoskeletal Disorders and Workplace Factors. A Critical Review of Epidemiologic Evidence for Work-related Musculoskeletal Disorders of the Neck, Upper-extremity, and Low Back. Cincinnati, OH: NIOSH, 1997.

Nordin M 2000 International society of the study of the lumbar spine presidential address: backs to work: some reflections. Spine 26 (8): 851-856, 2001.

Picavet HJS, Vlaeyen JWS, Schouten JSAG. Pain catastrophizing and kinesiophobia: predictors of chronic low back pain. Am J Epidem 158 (11): 1028-34, 2002.

Pincus T, Burton K, Vogel S, Field AP. A systematic review of psychological factors as predictors of chronicity/disability in prospective cohorts of low back pain. Spine 27 (5): E109-E120, 2002.

Ropponen A, Silventoinen K, Svedberg P, et. al. Health-related risk factors for disability pensions due to musculoskeletal diagnoses: a 30-year Finish twin cohort study. Scand J Public Health 39 (8): 839 – 48, 2011.

Ropponen A, Silventoinen K, Tynelius P, Rasmussen F. Association between hand grip/body weight ratio and disability pension due to musculoskeletal disorders: a population-based cohort study of 1 million Swedish men. Scand J Public Health 39 (8): 830-8, 2011.

Sivertsen B, Overland S, Neckelmann D, et. al. The long-term effect of insomnia on work disability: the Hunt-2 historical cohort study. Am J Epidem 163 (11): 1018 – 24, 2006.

Spitzer WO, LeBlanc FE, Dupuis M, et al: Scientific Approach to the Assessment and Management of Activity-related Spinal Disorders. Spine 12 (7S), 1987.

Spitzer WO, Skovron ML, Salmi LR, Cassidy JD, et al. Scientific monograph of the Quebec task force on whiplash-associated disorders: redefining 'whiplash' and its management. Spine 20 (8S), 1995.

Turner JA, Franklin G, Fulton-Kehoe D, et. al. Early predictors of chronic work disability: a prospective, population-based study of workers with back injuries. Spine 33 (25): 2809-2818, 2008.

Vandenbroucke JP, von Elm E, Altman DG, Gøtzsche PC, Mulrow CD, Pocock SJ,Poole C, Schlesselman JJ, Egger M; STROBE initiative. Strengthening the Reporting of Observational Studies in Epidemiology (STROBE): explanation and elaboration. Ann Intern Med. 2007 Oct 16;147(8):W163-94. PMID: 17938389

Vingard E, Nachemson A. Work-related Influences on Neck and Low Back Pain. In. Nachemson AL, Jonsson E. Neck and Back Pain: The scientific evidence of causes, diagnosis, and treatment. Lippincott Williams & Wilkins, Philadelphia, 2000: 97-126.

3 RESEARCH & DIAGNOSTIC TESTING (ACTIVITY-RELATED MSD)

Musculoskeletal healthcare is fully engaged in the modern era of evidence-based practice; the DRS© embraces the importance of this movement with a healthy dose of skepticism – no matter how strong the evidence there are limitations in applicability to individual patients. Our position is that internal evidence (i.e. objective assessment of the response of a patient to your treatment) ultimately trumps external evidence (i.e. strength of scientific evidence) in clinical practice.

An excellent overview of how to seek and use evidence can be found by reviewing the 2011 Oxford Center for Evidence-Based Medicine Levels of Evidence (Howick 2011 a, b; OCEBM 2011). You need to read the introduction and background documents before going to the 2011 table that explains and grades five levels of evidence. These five levels in descending order are: 1) systematic review, 2) randomized trial, 3) cohort study, 4) case series, 5) mechanistic reasoning.

Although this hierarchy correctly ranks the strength of the science the report recognizes that studies of lesser design can provide better evidence. And the level of evidence never suffices for good judgment and clinical experience. The OCEBM report suggests that you ask the following upon assessing the evidence: a) is your patient similar to the patients in the studies you've assessed, b) do the treatment benefits outweigh the harms, c) is there another treatment that is better, and d) are the patient's values and circumstances compatible with the treatment?

Similarly Malmivaara et. al. (2006) provided tools to evaluate the "applicability and clinical relevance of results in RCT" related to the study of spinal disorders. They used an assessment of the literature related to exercise therapy for LBP as an example to help clinicians become more critical readers. They asked five simple questions:

1. Are the patients described in detail so that you can decide whether they are comparable to those that you see in your practice?
2. Are the interventions and treatment settings described well enough so that you can provide the same for your patients?
3. Were all clinically relevant outcomes measured and reported?
4. Is the size of the effect clinically important?
5. Are the likely treatment benefits worth potential adverse effects?

Lastly, there are published standards for assessing the design and the conduct of scientific investigations and a system for rating any subsequent clinical guidelines. The clinician can use these standards and the rating system as a means of assessing scientific rigor and evidence:

*   STARD statement (Standards for the reporting of diagnostic accuracy studies) – STARD-statement.org
*   CONSORT statement (Consolidated standards of reporting trials) – CONSORT-statement.org
*   PRISMA statement (Preferred reporting items for systematic reviews and meta-analysis) – PRISMA-statement.org
*   STROBE statement (Strengthening the reporting of observational studies in epidemiology) – STROBE-statement.org
*   Kavanagh BP. The GRADE system for rating clinical guidelines. PLOS Medicine 6 (9): 1 – 5, 2009.

Reliability & Validity

Most musculoskeletal treatments are based on establishing a diagnosis or classifying (categorizing) the patient so they can be matched to a specific treatment protocol or approach. This is critical for clinical trials investigating treatment efficacy that involve homogenous group of patients, otherwise accurate comparisons cannot be made. To do this effectively we must know that the diagnosis or classification is reliable and accurate. As clinicians we need to be familiar with basic research methodology and capable of distinguishing quality and strength of evidence.

The treatment process starts with the history and physical examination, so the first step in clinical research is to investigate the accuracy of these procedures. Once established the accuracy of the diagnosis or classification system utilized to select the treatment approach can be investigated; once validity is established the efficacy of treatment can be investigated amongst a homogenous group of patients by a randomized controlled trial (RCT).

To establish diagnostic accuracy you must first prove reliability (both intra and inter-tester) and then validity (accuracy) of the examination or test procedure; this requires a proven gold standard for test comparisons. Bear in mind that there are issues with supposed 'gold standards' for musculoskeletal diagnostic studies, as the gold standard used can significantly affect diagnostic accuracy (Bachmann 2005). As previously mentioned, the STARD Statement (**STA**ndards for the **R**eporting of **D**iagnostic accuracy studies) serves as a checklist that clinicians can use to evaluate the strength of evidence relating to diagnostic accuracy (Bossuyt 2003; 2004).

1.   **Reliability** – this research identifies the consistency (stability) of the results or findings of examination and diagnostic procedures or tools. Good reliability means that the procedure or tool yields a consistent measurement when performed repeatedly by an individual (intra-rater reliability) and between individuals (inter-rater reliability); i.e. has a low rate of error. This does not mean that it measures what it intends to, nor does this prove it to be useful and effective. All it means is that it is reproducible for accuracy (validity) testing. The kappa coefficient (k) or intraclass correlation coefficient (ICC) are the statistics most commonly used to report the result of reliability studies:

Kappa coefficient (k) - this is the most commonly used measure of agreement after chance has been eliminated. This measure ranges from -1 (inverse relationship) to + 1 (direct relationship), with 0 indicating no relationship.

Intraclass correlation coefficients (ICC) - are used when the procedure involves interval or ratio measurements.

Table 3-1: the degree of reliability is determined by the kappa or ICC score.	
Good reliability	> 0. 75
Moderate reliability	0.50 – 0.75
Poor reliability	< 0.50
Acceptable reliability	Can be determined by the study; should be scrutinized by the reader.

2.   Validity – validity refers to the accuracy of the examination or diagnostic test procedure. As previously mentioned, validity studies require a gold standard to identify (rule-in) or rule-out the targeted disease or disorder. Validity studies determine the diagnostic power of the test; i.e. its predictive value, sensitivity, specificity, and likelihood ratio. This process starts with the use of a 2 X 2 contingency table, as follows (Table 3-2):

Table 3-2: A 2 x 2 contingency table compares the results of examination or diagnostic procedure to that of a 'Gold Standard' procedure (i.e. one with the greatest proven reliability and accuracy). The analysis starts by calculation of the true and false positive and negative rates, proceeds to predictive values, followed by sensitivity and specificity of the procedure. From there the likelihood ratios can be calculated and the diagnostic power determined.

	Gold Standard # Positive	Gold Standard # Negative	
Diagnostic Test # Positive	**A** # True Positives	**B** # False Positives	**Positive Predictive Value (PPV)** A/A + B
Diagnostic Test # Negative	**C** # False Negatives	**D** # True Negatives	**Negative Predictive Value (NPV)** D/C + D
	Sensitivity A/A + C	**Specificity** D/B + D	

Accuracy = 100 % X (A + D)/(A+B+C+D)

(Accuracy = # of true positive & negative/total # tested)

The predictive value is the next attribute to evaluate. This can be positive, meaning that the patient does have the disease or disorder when the test findings are affirmed. Or, the predictive value can be negative, meaning that the absence of a test finding indicates that the patient does not have the disease or disorder. This information is obtained from the 2X2 contingency table with the following formula (i.e. row calculation):

Positive predictive value (PPV) = 100 % X A/(A+B)

(PPV = True-positive #/true-positive + false negative)

Negative predictive value (NPV) = 100 % X D/(C+D)
(NPV = True-negative #/false-positive + true-negative)

This leads to the evaluation of the sensitivity and specificity of the assessment test or procedure (i.e. a column calculation). The sensitivity represents the ability of the test or procedure to identify those patients that <u>do have</u> the disorder or disease in question (true positive rate). A highly sensitive test is effective for ruling-out a disorder or disease when negative, but <u>not</u> necessarily for ruling-in because it may have a high false-positive rate also.

Sensitivity = 100 % X A/(A+C)
(Sensitivity = True-positive #/true-positive + false-negative)

The specificity represents the ability of the test or procedure to identify those patients that <u>do not</u> have the disorder or disease in question (true-negative rate). A highly specific test is effective at ruling-in a disorder or disease when positive, but <u>not</u> necessarily for ruling-out because it may have a high false-negative rate also.

Specificity = 100 % X D/(B+D)
(Specificity = True-negative #/false-positive + true-negative)

The last basic evaluation of the diagnostic test or procedure is to determine the likelihood ratio (LR). This evaluates the tests ability to alter the pretest probability that the patient has the disease or disorder in question. This is accomplished by evaluating a comparison of the sensitivity and specificity results. The likelihood ratio can be positive or negative in accordance with what was described for predictive values.

Positive LR increases the probability that the target disorder or disease is actually present, i.e. increasing the diagnostic power of the test.

Positive LR = Sensitivity/(1-specificity)

A negative LR increases the probability that the target disorder or disease is actually absent, i.e. increasing the diagnostic power and confidence in the test findings.

Negative LR = (1-Sensitivity)/Specificity

Table 3-3: the power of the likelihood ratio is determined by how large the positive score is to rule-in and how small the negative score is for ruling-out.		
	Positive LR	Negative LR
General increased likelihood	> 1	< 1
High probability	> 10	0.1
Moderate probability	5 – 10	0.1 – 0.2
Low probability, possibly important	2 – 5	0.2 – 0.5
Unlikely	1 – 2	0.5 – 1.0

Nordin et. al. (2008), based on the work of Sackett and Haynes, describes four phases that examination and diagnostic tests must go through in the process of proving validity and efficacy, as follows:

- **Phase I:** the test results in affected patients are proven conclusively to differ from those in normal individuals.
- **Phase II:** patients with certain test results are proven to be more likely to have the target disorder.
- **Phase III:** the results must have been proven to distinguish patients with and without the target disorder among those in whom it is clinically sensible to suspect the disorder.
- **Phase IV:** patients undergoing the specific diagnostic test must have proven to fare better in their health outcomes than similar patients who have not been exposed to the test.

Phase IV is the ultimate goal for healthcare because if a diagnostic test is not required for an optimal outcome why bother? In addition to this, ask yourself a few commonsense questions about the utility and applicability of the study results:

1. Is the gold standard really a gold standard?
2. How strong is the evidence; i.e. the statistical significance, the number of studies performed (is it repeatable) and the number of subjects studied?
3. How likely are you to encounter the problem in clinical practice?
4. Are the procedure or tools useful and does its use make sense in daily practice?

5. Does the use of the procedure or tool make a difference in clinical effectiveness and efficiency and how does it affect patient self-efficacy?

Other Considerations

Confidence Intervals (CI) – this measurement is used to provide a more accurate indication of how the results of a study (sample) population might compare to the population at large - a 95% CI is the general standard. When the results yield a smaller interval, there is greater precision for the study's findings. Conversely, a large interval indicates less precision.

Odds Ratio (OR) – this measurement is used to assess probability of a relationship between two variables; commonly used in gambling activities (e.g. odds of win vs. lose). In healthcare research OR represents the probability that a factor under investigation can be associated with a certain risk or outcome. It should be reported with a 95% CI. An odds ratio of 1 indicates that the risk or outcome is equal in both the control and study groups; the larger the number the greater the probability.

Clinical Prediction Rules (CPR) – a growing number of physical therapy-related trials have utilized clinical prediction rules (CPR) to analyze diagnostic accuracy, prognosis and prediction of response to treatment (Fritz 2009). A CPR rule can be defined as; " a clinical tool that quantifies the individual contributions that various components of the history, physical examination, and basic laboratory results make towards the diagnosis, prognosis or likely response to treatment in an individual patient." (Laupacis 1997)

CPRs are particularly useful in complex situations where there are heterogeneous groups of problems that fall into a general grouping; i.e. syndromes and non-specific disorders. There are three steps to developing and testing a CPR: 1) creation or derivation of the rule, 2) testing or validation of the rule, and 3) the assessment of the impact of the rule on clinical behavior and results; i.e. the impact analysis.

Table 3-4: Laupacis et. al. 1997: Hierarchy of evidence for clinical prediction rules (1 = strongest)
Level 1 Rules that can be used in a wide variety of settings with confidence that they can change clinician behavior and improve patient outcomes: at least one prospective validation in a different population and one impact analysis, demonstrating change in clinician behavior with beneficial consequences.
Level 2 Rules that can be used in various settings with confidence in their accuracy: demonstrated accuracy in either one large prospective study including a broad spectrum of patients and clinicians, or validated in several similar smaller settings who differ from one another.
Level 3 Rules that clinicians may consider using with caution and only if patients in the study are similar to those in your clinical setting: these rules have been validated in only one narrow prospective sample.
Level 4 Rules that need further evaluation before they can be applied clinically: these CPRs have been derived but not validated or have only been validated in split samples, large retrospective databases, or by statistical techniques.

CPRs have been used in medicine for many years (Wasson 1985; Laupacis 1997; McGinn 2000) and have recently emerged in the Physical Therapy literature (Fritz 2009). These studies should be reviewed and given strong consideration to incorporate findings into clinical practice; however realize that this is a young area of research and results need to be challenged and reinvestigated thoughtfully and constructively.

Gold Standards for Musculoskeletal Examination - the gold standards for physical examination procedures are those tests that are designed to provoke (reproduce) the patient's relevant symptoms (Waddell 1982; Matyas 1985; Potter 1985; Nelson 1988; McCombe 1989; Viikari-Juntura 1989; Laslett 1994; Maher 1994; Sandmark 1995; Donahue 1996; Wainner 2003; Seffinger 2004; Nordin 2008). These are typically movements, positions, manual procedures or functional/activity tests and to be reliable and valid they need to be operationalized. The least reliable and valid assessment procedures turn out to be palpation and observation. This does not mean that palpation and observational procedures cannot be reliable and useful, but they do have to be placed in a correct perspective and sequence of the examination when attempting to identify the source of the symptoms. Carefully developed operational definitions can convert procedures previously found to be unreliable to reliable (Strendler et. al. 1997).

Keep in mind that there is a significant problem with the accuracy of many musculoskeletal diagnostic tests, particularly a high incidence of false positive tests (i.e. poor specificity). However, these same tests often have a low rate of false negative results (i.e. good sensitivity); therefore these tests are more effective to rule-out a diagnosis or disorder, but you need more information to rule-in. And, surprisingly many of these musculoskeletal testing procedures have not been adequately studied for inter-rater reliability. We address these issues more specifically for each musculoskeletal region in the assessment-treatment-prevention series.

Perspective

US healthcare is a major industry consuming 17.9% of GDP in 2011; in many small university-based cities healthcare employers are often the largest in the community. When potential profit, prestige and influence are significant the possibility of misuse and overuse of services and misrepresentations of research escalate. At the 10th International forum for primary care research on low back pain a warning was issued related to the role of the "LBP medical industrial complex" in the epidemic of chronic pain and disability (Pransky 2011).

Conflicts of interest, intentional and unintentional withholding of data and ghost writing are some of the possibilities to consider when money, power and ego are involved (DeAngelis 2008; Ross 2008; Kho 2009; Lo 2010; National Research Council 2010; Vaccaro 2011). This was exemplified in the recent problems identified with the published trials regarding the use of bone morphotrophic protein (BMP-2) for spinal fusion surgery (Carragee 2012; Fu 2013). This created quite a stir in the spine surgery community with a commitment to more diligence in the review of published trials going forward (Bono 2013; Weiner 2013).

These problems exist at all levels of healthcare and research and need to be considered when evaluating the evidence. Our approach advocates for the individual, one patient at a time, and stresses the importance of adopting a prevention-based paradigm (Rath 2013).

References Chapter 3

Bachmann LM, Jüne P, Reichenbach S, Ziswiler HR, Kessels AG, Vögelin E. Consequences of different diagnostic 'gold standards' in test accuracy research: carpal tunnel syndrome as an example. Internat J Epidemiol 34: 953-5, 2005.

Bono CM, Wetzel FT, et. al. Black, white, or gray: how different (or similar) are YODA and The Spine Journal reviews of BMP-2? 13: 1001 – 5, 2013.

Bossuyt PM, Reitsma JB, Bruns DE. Et. al. Towards complete and accurate reporting of studies of diagnostic accuracy: the STARD initiative. Radiology 226 (1): 24 -28, 2003.

Bossuyt PM, Reitsma JB, Bruns DE. Et. al. Towards complete and accurate reporting of studies of diagnostic accuracy: the STARD initiative. Family Practice 21 (1): 4 -10, 2004.

Carragee EJ, Baker RM, Benzel EC, Bigos SJ, et. al. A biologic without guidelines: the YODA project and the future of bone morphogenetic protein-2 research. The Spine J 12 (10): 877-80, 2012.

Cleland J Orthopaedic Clinical Examination: an evidence-based approach for physical therapists. Icon Learning Systems, Carlstadt, NJ, 2005.

DeAngelis CD, Fontannarosa PB. Impugning the integrity of medical science: the adverse effects of industry influence. JAMA 299 (15): 1833-35, 2008.

Fritz JM. Clinical prediction rules in physical therapy: coming of age? JOSPT 39 (3): 159-61, 2009.

Fu R, Selph S, McDonagh M, Peterson K, et. al. Effectiveness and harms of recombinant human bone morphogenetic protein-2 in spine fusion: a systematic review and meta-analysis. Annals Int Med 158 (12): 877-89, 2013.

Howick J, Chalmers I, Glasziou P, et. al. "The 2011 Oxford CEBM Evidence Levels of Evidence (Introductory Document)". Oxford Centre for Evidence-based Medicine. http://www.cebm.net/index.aspx?o=5653

Howick J, Chalmers I, Glasziou P, et. al. "Explanation of the 2011 Oxford CEBM Evidence Levels of Evidence (Background Document)". Oxford Centre for Evidence-based Medicine. http://www.cebm.net/index.aspx?o=5653

Kavanagh BP. The GRADE system for rating clinical guidelines. PLOS Medicine 6 (9): 1 – 5, 2009.

Kho ME, Duffett M, Willison DJ, Cook DJ, Brouvers MC. Written informed consent and selection bias in observational studies using medical records: systematic review. BMJ

2009;338:b866 doi:10.1136/bmj.b866.

Lang TA, Secic M. How to Report Statistics in Medicine: Annotated Guidelines for Authors, Editors, and Reviewers. Am College Physicians, Philadelphia, 1997.

Laslett M, William M: The reliability of selected pain provocation tests for sacroiliac joint pathology. Spine 19 (11): 1243-1249, 1994.

Laupacis A, Sekar N, Stiell IG. Clinical prediction rules: a review and suggested modifications of methologoicla standards. JAMA 277 (6): 488-94, 1997.

Lo B. Serving two masters – conflicts of interest in academic medicine. NEJM 362 (8): 669- 71, 2010.

Maher C, Adams R. Reliability of pain and stiffness assessments in clinical manual lumbar spine examination. Physical Therapy 74(9): 801-809, 1994.

Malmivaara A, Koes BW, Bouter LM, van Tulder MW. Applicability and Clinical Relevance of Results in Randomized Controlled Trials The Cochrane Review on Exercise Therapy for Low Back Pain as an Example. Spine 31 (13): 1405–09, 2006.

Matyas TA and Bach TM: The Reliability of Selected Techniques in Clinical Arthrometrics. Australian J Physiother 31 (5): 175-195, 1985.

McCombe PF, Fairbank JCT, Cockersole BC, et al: Reproducibility of Physical Signs in Low-Back Pain. Spine 14 (9): 908-918, 1989.

McGinn TG, Guyatt GH, Wyer PC et. al. Users' guides to the medical literature: XXII: how to use articles about clinical decision rules. JAMA 284 (1): 79-84, 2000.

National Research Council (2010). The Prevention and Treatment of Missing Data in Clinical Trials. Panel on handling missing data in clinical trials. Committee on national statistics, division of behavioral and social sciences and education. Washington, DC: The National Academies Press. (Free PDF download: http://www.nap.edu/catalog/12955.html)

Nelson RM: NIOSH Low Back Pain Atlas of Standardized Tests/Measures. US Department of Health and Human Services. Public Health service, Centers for Disease Control, National Institute for Occupational Safety and Health, Division of Safety Research, Morgantown, W. Va., December 1988.

Nordin M, Carragee EJ, Hogg-Johnson Sheilah, et. al. Assessment of Neck Pain and Its Associated Disorders: Results of the Bone and Joint Decade 2000-2010 Task Force on Neck Pain and Its Associated Disorders Spine 33(4S): S101-22, 2008.

OCEBM Levels of Evidence Working Group "The Oxford 2011 Levels of Evidence". Oxford Centre for evidence-Based Medicine. http://www.cebm.net/index.aspx?o=5653.

Pransky G, Borkan JM, Young AE, Cherkin DC. Are we making progress? The tenth international forum for primary care research on low back pain. Spine 36 (19): 1608-14, 2011.

Potter NA and Rothstein JM: Intertestor Reliability for Selected Clinical Tests of the Sacroiliac Joint. Phy Ther 65 (11): 1671-1675, 1985.

Rath W. Prevention strategies for activity-related spinal disorders: recalibrating your clinical tools. APTA Pre-conference workshop, Salt Lake City, UT, June 26, 2013. (free download available: http://duffyrath.com/physical-therapist-in-syracuse).

Ross JS, Hill KP, Egilman DS, Krumholz HM. Guest authorship and ghostwriting in publications related to rofecoxib: a case study of industry documents from rofecoxib litigation. JAMA 299 (15): 1800-12, 2008.

Sackett DL, Haynes RB. Evidence base of clinical diagnosis: the architecture of diagnostic research. BMJ 324(7336): 539-41, 2002.

Sandmark H, Nisell R. Validity of five common manual neck pain provoking tests. Scand J Rehabil Med 27: 131-6, 1995.

Seffinger MA, Najm WI, Mishra SI, et. al. Reliability of spinal palpation for diagnosis of back and neck pain: a systematic review of the literature. Spine 29 (19): E413-25, 2004.

Strender LE, Sjoblom A, Sundell K, Ludwig R, Taube A Interexaminer Reliability in Physical Examination of Patients With Low Back Pain Spine 22(7): 814-820, 1997.

Vaccaro AR. Author conflict and bias in research: quantifying the downgrade in methodology. Spine 36 (14): E895-96, 2011.

Viikari-Juntura E, Porras M, Laasonen EM. Validity of clinical tests in the diagnosis of root compression in cervical disc disease. Spine 14 (3): 253-7, 1989.

Waddell G, Main CJ, Morris EW, Venner RM, Rae P, Sharmy SH, Galloway H. Normality and reliability in the clinical assessment of backache. Br Med J 284: 1519-23, 1982.

Wainner RS, Fritz JM, Irrgang JJ, Boninger ML, DeLitto A, Allison S. Reliability and diagnostic accuracy of the clinical examination and patient self-report measures for cervical radiculopathy. Spine 28(1): 52-62, 2003.

Wasson JH, Sox HC, Neff RK, Goldman L. Clinical prediction rules: applications and methodological standards. NEJM 313 (13): 793-99, 1985.

Weiner BK, Hurwitz EL, Schoene ML, Carragee EJ. Moving forward after YODA. The Spine J 13 (9): 995-97, 2013.

4 PAIN DEFINITIONS

Pain is the number one reason patients seek healthcare for MSD; a complex phenomenon with multiple dimensions, meanings and clinical considerations. This is clearly illustrated by the current definition of pain according to the International Association for the Study of Pain (IASP); *"An unpleasant sensory and emotional experience associated with actual or potential tissue damage, or described in terms of such damage."* (Merskey & Bogduk 2002). Table 4-1 has a list of IASP definitions of pain terms that to be used with discipline in clinical practice.

Table 4-1: Pain terms and IASP definitions that can apply to assessment and treatment of MSD.

Allodynia - Pain due to a stimulus that does not normally provoke pain.

Analgesia - Absence of pain in response to stimulation which would normally be painful.

Anesthesia dolorosa - Pain in an area or region which is anesthetic.

Causalgia - A syndrome of sustained burning pain, allodynia, and hyperpathia after a traumatic nerve lesion, often combined with vasomotor and sudomotor dysfunction and later trophic changes.

Central pain - Pain initiated or caused by a primary lesion or dysfunction in the central nervous system.

Dysesthesia - An unpleasant abnormal sensation, whether spontaneous or evoked.

Hyperalgesia - Increased pain from a stimulus that normally provokes pain.

Hyperesthesia - Increased sensitivity to stimulation, excluding the special senses.

Hyperpathia - A painful syndrome characterized by an abnormally painful reaction to a stimulus, especially a repetitive stimulus, as well as an increased threshold.

Hypoalgesia - Diminished pain in response to a normally painful stimulus.

Hypoesthesia - Decreased sensitivity to stimulation, excluding the special senses.

Neuralgia - Pain in the distribution of a nerve or nerves.

Neuritis - Inflammation of a nerve or nerves.

Neuropathic pain - Pain caused by a lesion or disease of the somatosensory nervous system.

Central neuropathic pain - Pain caused by a lesion or disease of the central somatosensory nervous system.

Peripheral neuropathic pain - Pain caused by a lesion or disease of the peripheral somatosensory nervous system.

Neuropathy - A disturbance of function or pathological change in a nerve: in one nerve, mononeuropathy; in several nerves, mononeuropathy multiplex; if diffuse and bilateral, polyneuropathy.

Nociception - The neural process of encoding noxious stimuli.

Nociceptive neuron- A central or peripheral neuron of the somatosensory nervous system that is capable of encoding noxious stimuli.

Nociceptive pain - Pain that arises from actual or threatened damage to non-neural tissue and is due to the activation of nociceptors.

Nociceptive stimulus- An actually or potentially tissue-damaging event transduced and encoded by nociceptors.

Nociceptor - A high-threshold sensory receptor of the peripheral somatosensory nervous system that is capable of transducing and encoding noxious stimuli.

Noxious stimulus - A stimulus that is damaging or threatens damage to normal tissues.

Pain threshold - The minimum intensity of a stimulus that is perceived as painful.

Pain tolerance level - The maximum intensity of a pain-producing stimulus that a subject is willing to accept in a given situation.

Paresthesia - An abnormal sensation, whether spontaneous or evoked.

Sensitization - Increased responsiveness of nociceptive neurons to their normal input, and/or recruitment of a response to normally sub-threshold inputs.

Central sensitization- Increased responsiveness of nociceptive neurons in the central nervous system to their normal or sub-threshold afferent input.

Peripheral sensitization - Increased responsiveness and reduced threshold of nociceptive neurons in the periphery to the stimulation of their receptive fields.

Pain Location Definitions: More Accurate Use of Terminology Needed

We need to be careful with our use of terminology if we are to improve our reliability and accuracy in diagnosing MSDs; but also to improve our ability to accurately communicate. The topographic description of symptoms is a particular problem with activity-related spinal disorders (ARSD). This evidenced when a study investigating the reliability of the low back examination finds that examiners can't even agree as to whether or not the patient has low back pain (Nelson 1979). Bogduk

(2002) explains the problem is not using standardized definitions; low back pain is a nonspecific term that could indicate symptoms in lumbar, lower thoracic, loin or buttock regions. He goes on to indicate if the patient reports buttock pain and never had any symptoms in the lumbar region the likelihood of the source being the lumbar spine is minute. Similarly, the term radicular pain is often used when the patient simply has non-specific referred pain into the upper or lower limb. This can be a reason for unnecessary and unsuccessful epidural steroid injections – one can't expect that bathing the root in steroid is going to help when it is not the source of the symptoms.

In the clinic patients with MSDs present with one of three patterns of symptoms as described by location; 1) local pain, 2) somatic referred pain and 3) neuropathic pain (central, peripheral and radicular). The following definitions used throughout this book and the DRS in general are based on the IASP guidelines (Merskey & Bogduk 2002):

Lumbar spinal pain – felt from top of S1 to bottom of T12 and as far lateral as the erector spinae. Posterior pain lateral to the erector spinae is loin pain.

Sacral spinal pain – felt anywhere over the area of the sacrum.

Coccygeal pain – felt anywhere over the area of the coccyx.

Buttock pain – felt anywhere over the posterior and lateral surface of the ilium and ischium, lateral to the sacrum/coccyx extending to the greater trochanter.

Radicular pain – "pain perceived as arising in a limb (or trunk wall)….pain is lancinating in quality and travels along a narrow band."

Referred pain – "pain perceived as occurring in a region of the body topographically distinct from the region in which the actual source of the pain is located."

Cervical spinal pain – "Pain perceived as arising from anywhere within the region bounded superiorly by the superior nuchal line, inferiorly by an imaginary transverse line through the tip of the first thoracic spinous process, and laterally by sagittal planes tangential to the lateral borders of the neck."

"Cervical pain can be subdivided into *upper cervical pain* and *lower cervical pain* by subdividing the above region into two equal halves by an imaginary transverse plane. Additionally, pain located between the superior nuchal line and an imaginary transverse line through the tip of the second cervical spinous process can be qualified as *suboccipital pain*."

Thoracic spinal pain – felt from top of T1 to the bottom of T12 and as far lateral as the erector spinae. Posterior pain felt lateral to the erector spinae is **posterior chest wall** pain; pain felt in the scapula(e) is a common site of somatic referred pain arising from the cervical spine (Cloward 1959).

Radicular pain – "Pain perceived as arising in a limb or the trunk wall caused by ectopic activation of nociceptive afferent fibers in a spinal nerve or its roots or other neuropathic mechanisms"

"The pain is lancinating in quality and travels along a narrow band. It may be episodic, recurrent, or paroxysmal according to the causative lesion or any superimposed aggravating factors."

"Lesions that directly compromise the dorsal root ganglion mechanically or indirectly compromise the spinal nerve and its roots by causing ischemia or inflammation of the axons. Specific entities include:

1. Foraminal stenosis due to vertical subluxation of the intervertebral joint, osteophytes stemming from the zygapophyseal joint or intervertebral disk, buckling of the ligamentus flavum, or a combination of any of the above.
2. Foraminal stenosis due to miscellaneous disorders of the zygapophyseal joint such as articular fractures, slipped epiphysis, ganglion, joint effusion, and synovitis.

3. Prolapsed intervertebral disk acting mechanically as a space-occupying lesion that compromises axons.
4. Prolapsed intervertebral disc material that elicits an inflammatory reaction in the vertebral canal that secondarily produces inflammation of adjacent neural elements.
5. Radiculitis caused by inflammatory exudates leaking from an intervertebral disk in the absence of frank prolapsed.
6. Radiculitis caused by inflammatory exudates from a zygapophyseal joint.
7. Radiculitis caused by viral infection or post-viral inflammation of a dorsal root ganglion, e.g. herpes zoster and psotherpetic neuralgia.
8. Radiculitis due to arteritis.
9. Tabes dorsalis."

Definition of radiculopathy: "Objective loss of sensory and/or motor function as a result of conduction block in axons of a spinal nerve or its roots."

In the cervical spine the C6 and C7 root are the most commonly affected (i.e. C5-6 and C6-7 segments); followed by C8 and C5; however radicular pain with or without radiculopathy is infrequent in comparison to local and somatic referred pain. In the lumbar spine the L5 and S1 roots are most commonly affected, followed by L4 and L3 – rarely L1 or L2 (i.e. an immediate caution as psoas weakness can be a sign of serious pathology).

Classification by Duration – Important Distinction: Acute vs. Chronic

How long a painful condition has been present is an important distinguishing factor for the assessment, treatment and prevention of MSD and disability. The most important distinction is between acute and chronic pain, with subacute a transitional period between the two.

Acute pain applies to the initial stage of a painful musculoskeletal condition; that is commonsense and appears simple. This is simple when there has been a traumatic event; many definitions of acute pain indicate a sudden onset of severe pain. However, many MSD develop as a result of no specific incident or event, or develop while performing a normal activity and do not necessarily produce severe symptom intensity initially. Rather than focus on the intensity of the pain or the mechanism of onset, DRS utilizes the definition of acute provided in the QTF report which focuses on how long the symptoms have been present; i.e. acute pain is that which has been present for less than 1 week.

Chronic musculoskeletal pain is clearly defined by its duration; i.e. pain that persists beyond the normal and expected time required for normal healing and/or the natural history for the specific musculoskeletal injury or disorder. The QTF report identifies an aggressive definition for chronic pain; i.e. that which has been present for > 7 weeks. The International Association for the Study of Pain (IASP) recognizes 3 months as a convenient point of delineation for chronic pain, but indicates the 6-month mark as the preferred timeframe for research purposes (Merskey & Bogduk 2002).

When defined by duration, subacute pain becomes that which has lasted somewhere between the definition of acute and chronic; i.e. somewhere from > 1 week to less than 3 – 6 months. DRS prefers the QTF report definition of subacute (i.e. > 1 < 7 weeks); most patients seen for this length of time should be recovered or heading predictably towards recovery. When there is doubt of full recovery by this time the patient needs to be thoroughly reassessed to identify and address factors interfering with their recovery before the condition becomes chronic.

A common distinction between acute and chronic pain is how it behaves. Acute musculoskeletal pain has clear mechanical behavior; activities, postures, movements affect the pain for the better or worse. With chronic pain the correlation between pain flares and specific activities is often poor (Hackzell 2004). Too often the patient and/or clinician assume a negative correlation between activity and the chronic pain; this assumption can facilitate activity avoidance behaviors, a major problem in managing chronic pain and disability.

Loeser developed a conceptual model of pain (Table 4-2) many years ago that is useful for clinical management; in this model disability is a pain behavior that is often iatrogenic and that becomes legitimized (Fordyce 1989).

Table 4-2: Taken from Fordyce (1989) description of Loeser's conceptual model of pain.

Nociception	Pain	Suffering	Pain Behavior
Noxious stimulus (thermal, mechanical or chemical energy) activating specialized free nerve endings that may or may not be perceived as pain.	Refers to the perception or stimulus identification process; nociceptive stimuli may be perceived as not painful and non-nociceptive stimuli may be perceived as painful.	Refers to the emotional response associated with anticipation of threat to well-being or to the positive outcome of future events related to the identification of pain.	The actions of people when they are hurting or suffering; e.g. moaning, limping, seeking medication, avoiding activity etc.

The biopsychosocial model emerged in the 1970s as a tool to manage psychiatric disorders more effectively (Engle 1977). Waddell championed the adoption of this model for managing ARSD, winning a Volvo Award in 1987. Waddell and colleagues developed an illness model (Table 7) that is useful for understanding the clinical presentation of chronic pain patients.

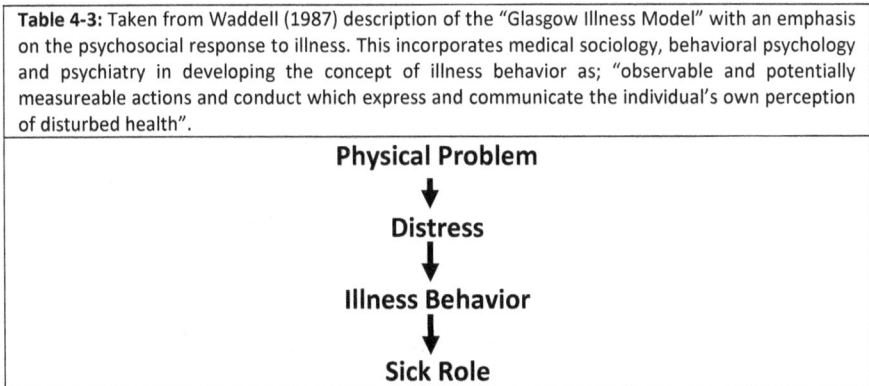

Table 4-3: Taken from Waddell (1987) description of the "Glasgow Illness Model" with an emphasis on the psychosocial response to illness. This incorporates medical sociology, behavioral psychology and psychiatry in developing the concept of illness behavior as; "observable and potentially measureable actions and conduct which express and communicate the individual's own perception of disturbed health".

Physical Problem

↓

Distress

↓

Illness Behavior

↓

Sick Role

Fordyce may have said it best in response to a research article published in Spine: "It is a marvel to me and a tribute to the persistence of selective attention that so many health care researchers seem unable to come to grips with what has been well known and repeatedly demonstrated: namely, that humans and the complex behaviors they emit can be understood only by considering their biomedical, genetic, psychological, and environmental/social contexts. To do less is to perpetuate a myth. Pain, particularly chronic low back pain, is transdermal. Put another way, perhaps pain ought to be seen as a verb, not a noun." (Fordyce 1999).

Chronic Widespread Pain is the modern term for the condition commonly called fibromyalgia. The point prevalence of this condition is reported to be as high as 11.2% (Croft et. al. 1993) and is second to osteoarthritis as the most common reason for a visit to the Rheumatologist (Arnold et, al. 2011). This disorder is frequently mislabeled a specific MSD when in actuality it is a nervous system disorder of unknown etiology. This group is characterized by an abundance of musculoskeletal symptoms with no significant objective physical examination (mechanical) findings to correlate to a specific MSD. In the DRS a function treatment strategy is employed for this group incorporating evidence for the efficacy of exercise (Busch et.a l. 2007).

The following is the 1990 criteria for this classification (Wolfe et. al. 1990):

1. History of widespread pain: Pain is considered widespread when all of the following are present and have been present for at least 3 months or longer: pain in the left side of the body, pain in the right side of the body, pain above the waist, and pain below the waist. In addition, axial skeletal pain (cervical spine or anterior chest or thoracic spine or low back) must be present. In this definition, shoulder and buttock pain is considered as pain for each involved side. "Low back" pain is considered lower segment pain.

2. Pain in ≥ 11 of 18 tender point sites on digital palpation: a tender point is considered positive only if the patient states that the palpation was painful, tender is not considered painful. Approximately 4 kg of pressure should be applied – see table 4-4 below.

This group of patients can effectively manage their disorder with a functional treatment paradigm, but not with the typical orthopaedic approach. These patients present with a disproportionate amount and severity of symptoms and little or no objective physical examination findings. When this group is misdiagnosed with an MSD label and treatment fails the patient is all too often blamed rather than initiating a close inspection of the accuracy of the diagnostic conclusion(s) and the appropriateness of the treatment strategy.

Table 4-4: The palpation sites used in the assessment for evidence of chronic widespread pain. There are 9 anatomical sites assessed bilaterally; ≥ 11 painful sites meets this component of the criteria for diagnosis. The presence of a second clinical disorder does not exclude the diagnosis of fibromyalgia. A modification of this classification has been published adding a measurement of symptom severity (Wolfe et. al. 2010) with mixed reviews and controversy.

Palpation Sites	Must be reported as painful with 4 kg of pressure
Occiput	bilateral, at the suboccipital muscle insertions.
Low Cervical	bilateral, at the anterior aspects of the intertransverse spaces at C5-C7.
Trapezius	bilateral, at the midpoint of the upper border.
Supraspinatus	bilateral, at origins, above the scapula spine near the medial border.
Second Rib	bilateral, at the second costochondral junctions, just lateral to the junctions on upper surfaces.
Lateral Epicondyle	bilateral, 2 cm distal to the epicondyles.
Gluteal	bilateral, in upper outer quadrants of buttocks in anterior fold of muscle.
Greater Trochanter	bilateral, posterior to the trochanteric prominence.
Knee	bilateral, at the medial fat pad proximal to the joint line.

Complex Regional Pain Syndrome (CRPS) is the modern name for what was previously called "Sudeck's atrophy" or "Reflex Sympathetic Dystrophy" (RSD), and "causalgia". There are two types of CRPS:

CRPS type 1 (RSD) – the onset of the associated symptom and sign complex after a minor injury or fracture of a limb.

CRPS type 2 (causalgia) - the onset of the associated symptom and sign complex after injury to a major peripheral nerve.

The following are common findings with CRPS (Charlton 2005):

Sensory signs and symptoms – constant burning in distal limb, disproportionate pain intensity to inciting event, allodynia and/or hyperalgesia, and sensory abnormalities most pronounced distally and not topographically associated to specific nerves.

Autonomic abnormalities – distal swelling, hyper or hypohidrosis, vasodilatation or vasoconstriction and skin temperature changes.

Trophic changes – abnormal nail growth, increased or decreased hair growth, fibrosis, thin/glossy skin and osteoporosis.

Motor abnormalities – weakness, coordination deficits, tremor, dystonia and neglect-like symptoms or symptoms of disturbed body perception of the affected extremity.

Kinesiophobia – Fear Avoidance Behaviors

Pain-related fear of activity or movement plays a major role in chronic musculoskeletal pain and disability (Crombez 1999; Fritz 2002; Picavet 2002; Al-Obaidi 2005; Lundberg 2011). Two objective tools to measure patient distress and fear avoidance behaviors have emerged over the past 20 years; 1) the fear-avoidance beliefs questionnaire or FABQ (Waddell 1992; 1993) and 2) the Tampa Scale for Kinesiophobia (Miller 1991). Not only are these questionnaires useful when assessing patients with chronic musculoskeletal pain, but they are sensitive to 'at risk' patients with acute pain (Swinkels-Meewisse 2003). The recognition of fear avoidance behaviors is highly relevant to developing an effective treatment strategy (George 2003; Childs 2004; Lundberg 2009). Physical Therapy has taken a leading role in this research.

Chronic Musculoskeletal Pain Neuroscience

Modern research has enlarged our understanding of pain, including identification of abnormal neurobiological and structural changes that occur in the central nervous system associated with chronic somatic pain. These pathological changes result in neural pathway dysfunction that causes an inadequate inhibitory and overactive excitatory processes (Clauw and Williams 2009). The term "central sensitivity syndrome" has been introduced to group this subset of patients (Yunus 2007; 2008). This field of research and practice provides a new and effective approach to chronic pain that is positive. In this context, psychosocial factors are viewed as a trigger (stressor) and not the cause – when adopted, this changes the mindset of the therapist and patient in regards to tactics for control. These are important clinical tools when guiding a patient with chronic pain back to activity and function.

Most clinicians need a sound scientific basis for their explanations to patients to have confidence in their approach. This can be difficult with chronic musculoskeletal pain when the symptoms and signs aren't consistent, are nonspecific and do not behave with mechanically predictive patterns. Mosley (2003) has championed methods to apply knowledge of the neurophysiology of chronic musculoskeletal pain that empowers the patient and can lead to effective, functional outcomes. An excellent overview of these concepts and guide for clinicians can be found in a recently published textbook by Louw and Puentedura (2013), entitled; "Therapeutic Neuroscience Education: Teaching Patients About Pain. A Guide for Clinicians." These concepts and the emerging evidence is very important to understanding our Functional Treatment Strategy. This strategy is utilized for patients with chronic musculoskeletal disorders that present with non-mechanical behavior of the pain where serious pathologies (i.e. contraindications to physical therapy) have been ruled-out.

References Chapter 4

Al-Obaidi SM, Beattie P, Al-Zoabi B, Al-Wekeel S. The Relationship of Anticipated Pain and Fear Avoidance Beliefs to Outcome in Patients With Chronic Low Back Pain Who Are Not Receiving Workers' Compensation. Spine. 30(9): 1051-1057, May 1, 2005.

Arnold LM, Clauw DJ, McCarberg BH. Improving the recognition and diagnosis of fibromyalgia. Mayo Clin Proc 86 (5): 457 – 64, 2011.

Bogduk N, McGuirk B. Pain Research and Clinical Management; Vol. 13: Medical Management of Acute and Chronic Low Back Pain. An Evidence-based Approach. Elsevier, Amsterdam, 2002.

Busch AJ, Barber KA, Overend TJ, Peloso PM, Schachter CL. Exercise for treating fibromyalgia syndrome. Cochrane Database Syst Rev. 2007 Oct 17: (4): CD003786.

Charlton JE (Editor). Core Curriculum for Professional Education in Pain, 3rd edition. IASP Press, Seattle, 2005.

Childs JD, Fritz JM, Flynn TW, Irrgang JJ, Johnson KK, Majkowski GR, Delitto A. A Clinical Prediction Rule To Identify Patients with Low Back Pain Most Likely To Benefit from Spinal Manipulation: A Validation Study. Ann Intern Med 141(12): 920-928, 2004.

Cloward, RB: Cervical Discography: A Contribution to the Etiology and Mechanism of Neck, Shoulder and Arm Pain. Ann Surg 150(6): 1052-1064, 1959.

Croft P, Rigby AS, Boswell R, Schollum J, Silman A. The prevalence of chronic widespread pain in the general population. J Rheumatology 20 (4): 710-13, 1993.

Crombez G, Vlaeyen JWS, Heuts PHTG, et al. Pain-related fear is more disabling than pain itself: evidence on the role of pain-related fear in chronic back pain disability. Pain 80:329–39, 1999.

Engle GL The need for a new medical model: A challenge for biomedicine. Science 196; 129-136, 1977.

Fordyce WE Learning factors in pain. Scand J Rheumatology Suppl [82]: 13-17, 1989.

Fordyce WE. Point of View (The effect of the Mensendieck exercise program as secondary prophylaxis for recurrent low back pain: a randomized, controlled trial with 12-month follow-up). Spine 24 (15): 1592, 1999.

Fritz JM, George SZ. Identifying psychosocial variables in patients with acute work-related low back pain: the importance of fear-avoidance beliefs. Physical Therapy 82 (10): 973-83, 2002.

George SZ, Fritz JM, Bialosky JE, Donald DA. The Effect of a Fear-Avoidance-Based Physical Therapy Intervention for Patients With Acute Low Back Pain: Results of a Randomized Clinical Trial. Spine. 28(23):2551-2560,2003.

Graven-Nielsen T, Arendt-Nielsen L, Mense S. Fundamentals of Musculoskeletal Pain. IASP Press, Seattle, 2008.

Guzman J, Hurwitz EL, Carroll LJ, Haldeman S, Côté P, Carragee EJ, Peloso PM, van der Velde G, Holm LW, Hogg-Johnson S, Nordin M, Cassidy JD. A New Conceptual Model of Neck Pain: Linking Onset, Course, and Care: The Bone and Joint Decade 2000-2010 Task Force on Neck Pain and Its Associated Disorders Spine 33(4S): S14-23, 2008.

Liszka-Hackzell JJ, Martin DP. An Analysis of the Relationship Between Activity and Pain in Chronic and Acute Low Back Pain Anesth Analg. 99:477-481, 2004.

Louw A, Puentedura E. Therapeutic neuroscience education: teaching patients about pain. A guide for clinicians. Internation Spine and Pain Institute, USA, 2013.

Lundberg M, Styf J, Jansson B. On what patients does the Tampa Scale for Kinesiophobia fit? Physiother Theory Pract 25 (7): 495-506, 2009.

Lundberg M, Frennered K, Hägg O, Styf J. The impact of fear-avoidance model variables on disability in patients with specific or nonspecific chronic low back pain. Spine 36 (19): 1547-53, 2011.

Main C, Wood P, Hollis S, et al. The distress and risk assessment method. A simple patient classification to identify distress and evaluate the risk of poor outcome. Spine. 17 (1):42–52, 1992.

Mayer EA, Bushnell MC, Editors. Functional Pain Syndromes: presentation and pathophysiology. IASP Press, Seattle, 2009.

Merskey H, Bogduk N, editors. Classification of chronic pain: descriptions of chronic pain syndromes and definitions of pain terms, 2nd ed. IASP Press, Seattle 2002.

Miller RP, Kori SH, Todd DD. The Tampa Scale. Unpublished report, Tampa, 1991.

Mosely GL A pain neuromatrix approach to patients with chronic pain. Manual Therapy 8 (3): 130-40, 2003.

Moseley GL. Unraveling the barrier to reconceptualization of the problem in chronic pain: the actual and perceived ability of patients and health professionals to understand the neurophysiology. J Pain 4 (4): 184-89, 2003.

Nelson MA, Allen MB, Clamp SE, et al: Reliability and Reproducibility of Clinical Findings in Low-Back Pain. Spine 4 (2): 97-101, 1979.

Picavet HSJ, Vlaeyen JWS, Schouten JSAG. Pain catastrophizing and kinesiophobia: predictors of chronic low back pain. Am J Epidemiol 156: 1028–34, 2002.

Swinkels-Meewisse EJCM, Swinkels RAHM, Verbeek ALM, Vlaeyen JWS, Oostendorp RAB. Psychometric properties of the Tampa Scale for Kinesiophobia and the fear-avoidance beliefs questionnaire in acute low back pain. Manual Therapy 8 (1): 29-36, 2003.

Waddell G: A new clinical model for the treatment of low-back pain: biopsychosocial. Spine 12 (7): 632-644, 1987.

Waddel G, Newton M, Henderson I, et al. A fear-avoidance beliefs questionnaire (FABQ) and the role of fear-avoidance beliefs in chronic low back pain and disability. Pain 52:157–68, 1993.

Wolfe F, Symthe HA, Yunus MB, Bennett R, Bombadier C. The American College of Rheumatology 1990 criteria for the classification of fibromyalgia. Arthritis Rheum 33: 160-72, 1990.

Wolfe, F., Clauw, D. J., Fitzcharles, M.-A., Goldenberg, D. L., Katz, R. S., Mease, P., Russell, A. S., Russell, I. J., Winfield, J. B. and Yunus, M. B. (2010), The American College of Rheumatology Preliminary Diagnostic Criteria for Fibromyalgia and Measurement of Symptom Severity. Arthritis Care & Research, 62: 600–610. doi: 10.1002/acr.20140

5 HISTORY-TAKING

The first step in the clinical assessment process is the patient history. This process identifies onset, duration, impact and correlation to previous injuries and problems. The history is when the relevant symptoms are identified, their behavior and impact on the patient is determined, and the functional goals are identified – critical to measuring the success of treatment. The history-taking process also initiates the therapeutic rapport with the patient and the process of looking for cautions and contraindications.

Table 5-1: Outline of the DRS Initial Evaluation Process (History & Basic Examination)
HISTORY
1. Preliminary Patient Information   1.1 Demographics   1.2 Billing Information   1.3 Medical/Surgical History/Cautions & Contraindications   1.4 Habits/goals for treatment
2. Pain & Function Questionnaires   2.1 Self-reported Symptom Location   2.2 Self-reported Symptom intensity & frequency   2.3 Self-reported Interference with ADL
3. History (Interview)   3.1 Occupation, Recreation, Activity Status   3.2 4- Key Questions: onset, symptom location, frequency & behavior   3.3 Imaging and Diagnostic Tests   3.4 Previous history, trauma and other questions   3.5 Establish Function/Activity Goals for Treatment

The History-Taking Process

The development of effective communication and interview skills is critical to the Duffy-Rath System©. The initial interview process is the first step to understanding the patient's disorder, how their problem has affected them and it initiates patient education and training for self-efficacy. At the end of the interview you should have an expectation for the physical examination, an understanding of the relevant biomechanical factors in the patient's lifestyle, and you have started to formulate a plan for the search for TTFB®. The response patterns that emerge during the interview guide and influence the clinical process. Your ability to remain disciplined and focused, yet pleasant and therapeutic, during this process is critical to success.

To make the history-taking and basic examination process efficient, reliable and accurate it needs to be standardized with sound operational definitions, and kept as simple as possible. When this is lacking then agreement on simple questions that are essential to diagnosis and treatment, no less research, are rendered unreliable. This was exemplified in a study of the reproducibility of clinical findings with low back patients when examiners could not even agree whether or not the patient had back pain (Nelson 1979); Bogduk (2002) cites this study as evidence for the need to use standardized and accepted definitions – in this example, the need to use the topographical definitions adopted by the IASP. And, in general it is important to keep the process as short and simple as possible to improve the chance of achieving good inter-examiner reliability (Myers et. al. 2011).

Patient Information and Preliminary Screening

The patient can provide a significant amount of information prior to coming to the office and/or entering the treatment room. This streamlines the therapist interview time with the patient, screens for cautions and contraindications, and enables the therapist to focus on key issues relevant to the patient's current problem, yet still be thorough. This information can be obtained online, emailed and/or completed while in the waiting room (Boissonnault 1994; 1999; 2005). We recommend obtaining the following information:

1. **Basic Demographics** – this includes age (DOB), occupation, gender, address etc.

2. **Case-type (method of payment)** – we refer to this as case-type; i.e. workers' comp, private insurance, MVA, gov't program, self-pay and other. In addition we identify whether or not the patient is currently seeing a chiropractor and/or has retained a lawyer to represent a claim.

3. **Reason for Treatment** – this identifies the body region(s) and whether or not the patient has received previous care for this episode; if so, what treatment has been received.

4. **Medical, Surgical & General Health Information** – this identifies height, weight (BMI can be calculated), heart rate, blood pressure, hand dominance, medical diagnoses (co-morbidities), previous surgeries, a statement of health, unexplained weight loss and prescription medications.

5. **Special Questions** – these questions are specific to the identification of cautions or contraindications to physical therapy treatment. The questions specifically target disorders affecting the cauda equina, spinal cord and vertebral-cerebral arteries.

6. **Exercise Habits** – this identifies the patient's current exercise and health habits that require consideration for short-term and long-term management.

7. **Authorizations** – consent for treatment and authorization to release information to the third party payer, HIPPA requirements, private payment agreement and/or release agreements for research or teaching purposes (presented and signed at the office).

8. **Goal for Treatment** – in the patient's own words, why has he/she come to you for treatment?

Note: The therapist should always review this information with the patient prior to starting the history, seeking qualification of information provided and making certain important information was not omitted and/or that what was provided is accurate. Ask the patient to come to the first appointment 15 - 20 minutes prior to the scheduled starting time if filling this out in the office.

Pain & Function Questionnaires

Tools to measure pain and perceived (self-rated) functional ability have become a mainstay in clinical practice. When we first developed the Duffy-Rath Questionnaire (DRQ) in 1987 most of our colleagues thought this was asking too much of the patients, predicting they would stop coming for treatment. This prediction was proven incorrect; measuring this status at each treatment session was invaluable. These questionnaires are not only useful for outcome assessment, but help with patient management during the course of treatment. Whatever tools you choose to use be certain to review the questionnaire with the patient so that they understand how to answer the questions, and train your front office staff to provide guidelines and instructions to the patient.

Pain Measurements – there are many tools to measure pain, our focus is to three dimensions: 1) location, 2) intensity and 3) frequency.

Pain (symptom) location is classically measured by means of a pain drawing. In general the location of symptoms can be described as local, somatic referred, radicular or neuropathic, and widespread. Pain location with MSD usually shrinks (contracts or centralizes) as the condition improves; increases (expands or peripheralizes) as the condition worsens. Ransford et. al. (1976) found that there was good correlation between the pain drawing and the MMPI in low back pain patients; possibly providing early indication of relevant psychosocial factors.

Pain (symptom) intensity is the most common pain measure. The visual analogue scale (VAS) and the numeric rating scale (NRS) are the two gold standards (von Korff 2000, Wainner 2003; Nordin 2008). The difference between the two is that the VAS has a 10 cm line anchored on one end with no pain and the other with worst pain possible; the NRS has the same anchors with 0 (no pain) at one end and 10 (worst possible) at the other. Ostelo et. al. (2008) indicates that ≥ 30% improvement is required for a significant clinical change. Turner et. al. found that pain intensity ratings were not as predictive of work disability as are the severity of self-rated functional questionnaires.

In general **pain (symptom) frequency** has been an overlooked pain measure; however this is a very important component of pain assessment for clinical management strategies. We developed a NRS for pain frequency with 0 = not present at any time to 10 = always present. This has not been investigated for reliability or validity. The importance of symptom frequency is explored in detail as one of the 4 key interview (history-taking) questions.

Self-reported Function Questionnaires

Self-rated functional ability has become an important outcome measure for MSD and can be an early predictor of work disability with low back pain patients (Turner 2008). The most reliable and validated tools are region specific; i.e. low back, neck, upper limb, lower limb etc. There are so many questionnaires available that outcome comparisons can be difficult or impossible (Deyo 1998). The following are some of the most reliable, validated and responsive questionnaires used for self-rated functional ability with ARMSD:

1. **Low Back** – the Oswestry Disability Index and the Roland Morris Disability Questionnaire (Fairbank 1980, 2000; Roland 1983, 2000; Deyo 1998).
2. **Neck** – the Neck Disability Index (Riddle 1998; Nordin 2008) with consideration to the Patient Specific Functional Scale (Cleland 2006).
3. **Upper extremity** – there are no clear gold standard questionnaires for the upper limb (Fayad 2004; 2005). Currently accepted tools include: Nordic Musculoskeletal Questionnaire, the Upper Extremity Questionnaire, the Neck and Upper Limb Instrument, the Patient-Specific Functional Scale, the modified DASH-9, the Shoulder Pain and Disability Index (Salerno 2002; Paul 2004; MacDermid 2006; Gabel 2009;Hill 2011)
4. **Lower extremity** – as with the upper limb the issue of gold standards is in question. Currently accepted tools include: the Lower Extremity Functional Scale, the Activities of Daily Living Scale, the Hip Disability and Osteoarthritis Outcome Score, Harris Hip Score, the Oxford Hip Score, the Lysholm Knee Scale, the Tegner Activity Scale, Cincinnati Knee Rating System, Foot Function Index the Sports Ankle Rating System, the Foot and Ankle Ability Measure, the Foot Function Index and the Patient-Specific Functional Scale (Irrgang 1998; Nilsdotter 2003; Swinkels 2004; Hart 2005; Martin 2007; van der Martijn 2008; Pua 2009; Wang 2010).

Standardized Musculoskeletal Assessment Forms

Standardized forms for recording the patient history that have clear guidelines and definitions improve the reliability and accuracy of the information obtained and the ability to communicate with colleagues within and outside of your practice setting. As a general rule you should keep the process as short and simple as possible, focusing to questions that are most relevant to getting at root cause(s) and understanding the behavior and effect of the problem on the patient's ability to be active and to function.

Before beginning the history interview explain the whole assessment process to the patient. Let the patient know that you are going to follow a structured list of questions designed to help figure-out how to solve their problem, so you are going to be focused on obtaining answers to each question (or identify that there is no answer). However, reassure them that at the end of the interview they will be provided the opportunity to tell you more if they feel that anything has been overlooked (i.e. this is important as it often puts the patient at ease knowing they will have this opportunity if needed).

The history portion of the standardized assessment form should have four components; 1) demographics, 2) key questions, 3) other questions and 4) functional/activity goals.

1. **Patient Demographics** – this should include the name, age, referring physician (when not applicable identify the family physician), occupation, recreational activities and the date. We have found that it is very important to identify the patient's activity status at the time of the initial assessment; i.e. active (working full duty, normally active), restricted (work or normal activities restricted), or idle (not working because of their MSD or avoiding > 50% of normal ADL). This is predictive of the need for more visits and weeks on program to achieve functional goals and an increased likelihood that the symptoms will not be totally eliminated, but instead may be only controlled so as not to interfere with restoration of activity tolerance; i.e. a patient that has become inactive as a result of their MSD predictably requires more visits to achieve a good (not excellent) outcome (see Table 5-2 below).

The last bit of information obtained from demographics is the physical demands of the patient's occupation and recreational activities. This is important for designing a target-specific, individualized treatment and long-term plan and critical to our concept of strategic strength and conditioning to prevent recurrence. Once demographics are obtained the actual interview begins by seeking the answers to 4 key questions.

Activity Status	Excellent	Good	Fair	Poor	Mean Visits	Mean Weeks
Active	59.2 %	29.6 %	5.8 %	5.4 %	5.2 visits	4.4 weeks
Idle	41.0 %	29.5 %	16.7 %	12.8 %	9.8 visits	6.8 weeks

Table 5-2: Our first outcome study was a consecutive case-series outcome study (N=455) of ARSD patients seen in our clinic in New Jersey (i.e. the 'Spine Center Study'). 319 patients met our inclusion criteria for an ARSD, and we found that the patient's activity status at the time of the initial evaluation (active or idle) had a significant effect on effectiveness and efficiency of treatment. This has been a consistent finding with our internal evidence studies ever since.

2. The DRS 4 Key Questions – these four questions provide the most relevant information for the Duffy-Rath System©. Patients with previous episodes and those with chronic conditions need to be focused to the current episode, and to the current behavior of their problem.

Be pleasant and let your interest in helping to solve the problem shine through. Remain focused and disciplined to the process so that you obtain accurate and relevant information. Make certain that the patient understands the questions, and answers the question that has been asked – realize that a patient's inability to answer a question is an answer and a relevant clinical finding.

Key Question # 1: Onset Information

This first question has 2 components: first establish when this episode started (i.e. date of onset), and then how it started (mechanism of onset).

Date of onset: It is best to establish the onset date for the current ARSD first. On our assessment form you find a section to record either the actual date (month/day/year) or an estimated date (+/-, record month and year) when the patient cannot identify an actual one. I have found that more patients provide estimated dates.

When patients are having difficulty estimating when the current ARSD started, ask them to identify the last time they felt and functioned normally in regards to the region of their ARMSD; i.e. no symptoms and no interference with their normal activities for a week or longer. The month and year is then recorded in the estimated section.

Some patients have frequently repeating acute disorders; i.e. they are completely normal in between episodes. Some have not returned to normal for a long period of time, but have episodic exacerbations. The clinical expectation for these two groups of patients is different, but they are easily confused as the same when the history-taking process is sloppy.

Duration of disorder - based upon the QTFR (Spitzer et. al. 1987), we categorize the duration of the episode:

Acute – less than 7 days
Subacute - one to seven weeks
Early chronic – 7 – 26 weeks
Late chronic - > 26 weeks

The Mechanism of Onset: How did this episode start? Once the onset date is established ask the patient; "how did the episode start; i.e. was there one incident or event you can identify that caused the symptoms to commence?"

NIE – there is no one incident or event.
Incident-A – this is an incident related to a normal activity of daily living (ADL).
Incident-B – this is an unguarded, unexpected, sudden biomechanical component of force that occurred with a normal ADL (e.g. slipped but did not fall).
Trauma – there was a high velocity, high magnitude accident ± impact (e.g. motor vehicle accident, fall, struck by an object etc.).

Once the mechanism has been established, identify any relevant biomechanical and physiological factors associated with the onset when possible. When there was NIE ask the patient what they think might have been relevant factors, or if there were any unusual physical activities performed in the immediate days before the symptoms developed? This is recorded on the line provided for this information.

Table 5-3: Mechanism of onset study: we performed a prospective study of the mechanism of onset for 1,326 consecutive patients referred to one of our onsite industrial clinics. The mechanism for onset was placed into one of 4 groups following operative definitions: 1) NIE – no specific incident or event, 2) Incident A – performing a normal ADL (e.g. sitting, bending over, lifting something normal, reaching etc.), 3) Incident b – a sudden, unguarded force with a normal ADL (e.g. slipped walking but did not fall, lowering a box and it slipped and tried to catch it etc.), and 4) Trauma – car accident, fall, struck by something etc.

Category	NIE	Incident - A	Incident - B	Trauma	Total
Overall	690	345	128	158	1321
Population %	52.2	26.1	9.7	12.0	100
Work-related	462	295	109	103	969
Group %	47.7	30.4	11.2	10.7	100
Not Work-related	228	50	19	55	352
Group %	64.8	14.2	5.4	15.6	100

Patients with NIE or incident-A as the mechanism of onset fall into the cumulative strain disorder (CSD) group, indicating biomechanical and physiological habits are at the root cause. Vulnerability to incident-B onsets is influenced by habits (i.e. Wolf's Law) but are not the root cause; trauma is clearly an accident, consequently a safety issue for prevention with treatment guided by known stages of healing and the specifics of the injury.

Key Question # 2: Symptom Location

Symptoms are a report by the patient of what they feel, and the location is where they feel it. The symptoms may be in one isolated spot only (i.e. local), radiating in a non-specific pattern (i.e. somatic referred) or radicular (narrow band in the limb of severe intensity following a nerve root distribution, accompanied by nerve root signs) – see table 5-4 below. Multiple sites or locations of symptoms can be due to one lesion, or multiple lesions presenting simultaneously.

Each area of symptoms needs to be isolated and then investigated individually with the remaining key questions used to determine this. Once I identify that the current location of symptoms is possibly due to multiple problems presenting simultaneously, I number the different locations (e.g. #1 = across lumbar spine, # 2 = lateral buttock, # 3= P-L thigh and calf etc.) to see if they have the same or differing frequencies and behavior.

The location of the symptoms at onset and those present currently need to be isolated and identified. The current symptoms are the most important for the assessment process and initiation of treatment.

At onset – where were the symptoms first felt? Provides information about likely mechanics of onset if there was no incident or event, and the most likely source of the symptoms; e.g. pain felt initially in the center of the lumbar spine is coming from a mid-line structure and the forces involved are symmetrical in the sagittal plane.

Current – establish where the symptoms have been felt recently (past week, or couple weeks if a chronic problem). If there are radiating symptoms establish the most severe (predominant), a general description (aching, sharp, burning, numbness, tingling etc.) and symmetry. This is the most important symptom location question for the assessment process, developing a treatment strategy and measuring results.

Other (PRN) – describe any other symptoms when applicable.

	QTF 1 Local Pain	QTF 2 Local + prox. referred	QTF 3 Local + distal referred	QTF 4 Radicular
Table 5-4: In our first outcome study more than 80% of the patients seen for physical therapy treatment had a nonspecific back or neck pain disorder (QTF 1-3). This is consistent with the literature that indicates 70 – 90 % of ARSD are nonspecific. QTF = Quebec Task Force (Spitzer 1987)				
Spine Center study (N = 319)	122 38.3 %	58 18.2 %	85 26.6 %	54 16.9 %

Key Question # 3: Symptom Frequency

Symptom frequency is a measure of severity and behavior. When symptoms are the product of a nociceptive stimulus, the cause is mechanical (i.e. deformation, distortion of innervated tissue), chemical (i.e. inflammation or aggregation of noxious agents), or thermal (not applicable to our discussion). When the nociceptive stimulus increases the symptoms become more frequent to the point where they are continuous (i.e. larger concentrations of chemicals or constant mechanical distortion or distention). However, the perception of pain does not require a nociceptive stimulus and this is frequently the case with chronic pain, especially chronic widespread pain or neuropathic pain (central or peripheral).

Constant symptoms: the symptoms are continuous and never 'shut-off' or feel completely normal (i.e. never rated as 0). These symptoms are labeled **'mechanical constant'** when the intensity of these symptoms increase and decrease with activities, movements and positions. These symptoms are labeled **'non-mechanical constant'** when the intensity of these symptoms does not alter in response to activities, movements or positions.

Intermittent: the symptoms are intermittent when they at least temporarily stop, 'turn-off', drop to 0 or feel normal for time periods during the day. These symptoms are labeled **'stable intermittent'** when they quickly or immediately cease when the patient stops doing whatever it is that triggered them and there is no activity-related consequence as a result. The symptoms are labeled **'unstable intermittent'** when the patient stops the triggering activity and the symptoms persist, have consequences and/or progressively increase with additional exposure.

Non-mechanical constant pain is very concerning and requires careful clinical attention as this is characteristic of a medical and possibly sinister condition – this requires further work-up and you should confer with the patient's medical physician. Mechanical constant and unstable intermittent pain requires a conservative and careful approach to both examination and treatment so that the patient's condition is not irritated – not a good way to gain patient confidence. Stable intermittent symptoms require a thorough mechanical assessment.

Remember that you need to determine the frequency for each of the symptom location patterns identified with key question 2 when there is more than one.

Key Question # 4:   Symptom Behavior (Current)

This is a critical and unique section of the history-taking. This line of questioning addresses the presence or absence of mechanical patterns of symptom behavior, identifies what ADL are interfered with by the disorder (remember to compare to the DRQ), provides insight into the patient's objectivity, shows your determination to get to root causes of the problem and is frequently very educational.   Explain the process to the patient before you begin.

Table 5-5: Standardized terms used to describe symptoms response to assessment and/or treatment procedures.	
Term	**Definition**
Better	The activity/position reduces or abolishes symptoms that were present.
Worse	The activity/position produces symptoms that were not present, or increases those that were present.
Varies	The effect upon the symptoms varies. Have the patient explain this and/or ask more questions to learn more. This is a common and very important response as you and the patient will learn a great deal of relevant information.
No Effect (NE)	If symptoms are present the activity/position will not increase or decrease them. If symptoms are not present, the activity/position does not produce any effect.
Don't Know/Not Sure (???)	Haven't performed the activity/position recently, have not paid attention or am not sure.

Four groups of questions:

- **The effect of specific ADL on the symptoms** – this is the bulk of the questioning; adjust the questions to activities, movement and positions relevant to the region of the musculoskeletal disorder. Be certain to note what symptoms are affected, in what sequence (when applicable) and anything that is biomechanically specific to the response of the symptoms.
- **Effect of time of day** – this is a more general line of questioning, looking to see if the symptoms are their best or worst at certain time periods, or are they a product of specific activities/positions regardless of day time.
- **Val Salva's/deep breath** – this is most relevant to spinal disorders; pain upon coughing, sneezing or straining is not pathognomic, but highly associated with discal pathology. Pain and difficulty taking a

deep breath with thoracic spinal pain is strongly associated with a relevant loss of segmental thoracic extension.

- **Other** – always give the patient an opportunity to provide more information that your structured process and approach may not have uncovered.

3.   **Diagnostic Tests:**   determine what diagnostic tests and procedures have been performed this episode. Determine if the radiographic analysis is complete, or is more information required. Ask the patient to report the results, and compare this to a review of the official diagnostic reports. Look for the impact that the results of these tests and the explanations provided have had on the patient's perception of the problem. Most importantly, come to a conclusion as to whether or not the results of the diagnostic test are relevant to the patient's signs, symptoms and activity dysfunction (Bedson 2008). We covered the problems with the diagnostic accuracy of musculoskeletal imaging – potentially this will improve when these can incorporate movement and biomechanical loading to look for anatomical change and presence or absence of correlation to symptom change; i.e. kinetic imaging (Zou 2008).

4. Previous History & Treatment: Determine if this is a recurrent problem or not. If so, how frequent and is this episode similar to previous ones? What treatment have they had in the past, and what was their response to these treatments?

5.   Accidents/Trauma: Ask about significant accidents or trauma that could relate to the diagnosis and problem, and/or influence treatment.

6.   Other Questions: The very last question of the history, prior to setting functional goals, is to ask if there is anything else to report, or overlooked in the history thus far. This is important, as the structured interview doesn't always capture all the relevant information.

7.   Setting Functional Goals – you and the patient will establish 2 – 3 functional (activity) goals for treatment. These should be normal ADL tasks that the patient's problem has interfered with, or he/she are currently unable to perform. These were identified during the assessment of the current behavior of the symptoms. Once the function goals are established, eliminating or decreasing interference with these ADL tasks becomes the goal of the treatment program, and a measure of its success.

The W.H.O. has adopted the International Classification of Functioning, Disability and Health (ICF) Model to measure health and disability. This model stresses the importance of objectifying function and placing the ability of the individual to meet those demands within the context of their environmental and societal factors. This is evidence of the influence and evolution of the BioPsychoSocial model in healthcare. The following is the flowchart for ICF:

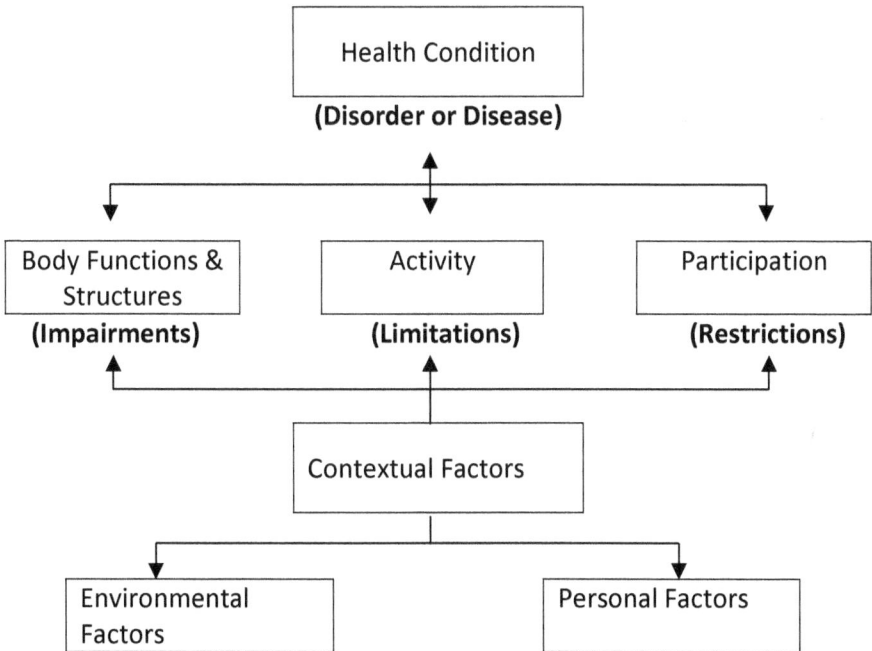

```
                    ┌─────────────────────────┐
                    │    Health Condition     │
                    │  (Disorder or Disease)  │
                    └─────────────────────────┘
                               ▲
        ┌──────────────────────┼──────────────────────┐
        ▼                      ▼                      ▼
┌─────────────────┐  ┌─────────────────┐  ┌─────────────────┐
│ Body Functions &│  │    Activity     │  │  Participation  │
│   Structures    │  │                 │  │                 │
│  (Impairments)  │  │  (Limitations)  │  │  (Restrictions) │
└─────────────────┘  └─────────────────┘  └─────────────────┘
        ▲                      ▲                      ▲
        └──────────────────────┼──────────────────────┘
                    ┌─────────────────────────┐
                    │   Contextual Factors    │
                    └─────────────────────────┘
              ┌──────────────┴──────────────┐
              ▼                             ▼
    ┌─────────────────┐           ┌─────────────────┐
    │  Environmental  │           │ Personal Factors│
    │     Factors     │           │                 │
    └─────────────────┘           └─────────────────┘
```

References Chapter 5

Bedson J, Croft PR. The discordance between clinical and radiographic knee osteoarthritis: a systematic search and summary of the literature. BMC Musculoskel Disord 2008; 9:116.

Bogduk N, McGuirk B. Pain Research and Clinical Management; Vol. 13: Medical Management of Acute and Chronic Low Back Pain. An Evidence-based Approach.

Elsevier, Amsterdam, 2002.

Bogduk N, McGuirk B. Pain Research and Clinical Management: Pain Research and Clinical Management of Acute and Chronic Neck Pain. An Evidence-based Approach. Edinburgh, Elsevier, 2006.

Boissonnault WG, Koopmeiners MB. Medical history profile: orthopaedic physical therapy outpatients. JOSPT 20(1): 2–10, 1994.

Boissonnault WG. Prevalence of comorbid conditions, surgeries, and medication use in a physical therapy outpatient population: a multicentered study. JOSPT 29(9):506 –519, 1999. (discussion 520–525)

Boissonnault WG, Badke MB. Collecting health history information: the accuracy of a patient self-administered questionnaire in an orthopaedic setting. Physical Therapy 85(6):531-43, 2005.

Cleland JA, Fritz JM, Whitman JM, Palmer JA. The Reliability and Construct Validity of the Neck Disability Index and Patient Specific Functional Scale in Patients with Cervical Radiculopathy. Spine 31(5): 598-602, 2006.

Deyo RA, Battie M, Beurskens AJ, et al. Outcome measures for low back pain research. A proposal for standardized use. Spine 23(18): 2003-13, 1998.

Fairbank JCT, Davies JB, Mbaot JC, O'Brien JT. The Oswestry Low Back Pain Disability Questionnaire. Physiotherapy 66:271-3, 1980.

Fairbank JCT, Pyrsent PB. Oswestry Disability Index Spine 25(22):2940-53, 2000.

Fayad F, Mace Y, Lefeyre-Colau MM. Shoulder disability questionnaires: a systematic review. Ann Readapt Med Phy 2005 Jul: 48(6): 298-306. Epub 2005 Apr 26.

Fayad F, Mace Y, Lefeyre-Colau MM, Poiradeau S, Rannou F, Revel M. Measurement of shoulder disability in the athlete: a systematic review. Ann Readapt Med Phy 47(6): 389-95, 2004.

Gabel CP, Yelland M, Melloh M, Burkett B. A modified QuickDash-9 provides a valid outcome instrument for upper limb function. BMC Musculoskelet Disord 2009;10:161.

Hart DL, Mioduski JE, Stratford PW. Simulated computerized adaptive tests for measuring functional status were efficient with good discriminant validity in patients with hip, knee, or foot/ankle impairments. J Clin Epidemiol 58 (6): 629-38, 2005.

Hefford C, Abbott JH, Arnold R, Baxter GD. The patient-specific scale: validity, reliability, and responsiveness in patients with upper extremity musculoskeletal problems. JOSPT

42 (2): 56-65, 2012.

Hill CL, Lester S, Taylor AW, Shanahan ME, Gill TK. Factor structure and validity of the shoulder pain and disability index in a population-based study of people with shoulder symptoms. BMC Musculoskelet Disord 2011 Jan 12;12:8.

Irrgang JJ, Snyder-Mackler L, Wainner RS, Fu FH, Harner CD. Development of a patient-reported measure of function of the knee. JBJS 80A (8): 1132-45, 1998.

MacDermid JC, Solomon P, Prkachin K. The shoulder pain and disability index demonstrates factor, construct and longitudinal validity. BMC Musculoskelet Disord 2006 Feb 10;7:12.

Martin RL, Irrgang JJ. A survey of self-reported outcome instruments for the foot and ankle. JOSPT 37 (1):72–84, 2007

Myers HL, Thomas E, Hay EM, Dziedzic KS. Hand assessment in older adults with musculoskeletal hand problems: a reliability study. BMC Musculoskeletal Disorders 2011, 12:3 http://www.biomedcentral.com/1471-2474/12/3

Nelson MA, Allen MB, Clamp SE, et al: Reliability and Reproducibility of Clinical Findings in Low-Back Pain. Spine 4 (2): 97-101, 1979.

Nilsdotter AK, Lohmander LS, Klässbo M, Roos EM. Hip disability and osteoarthritis outcome score (HOOS) – validity and responsiveness in total hip replacement. BMC Musculoskel Disord 2003; 4:10.

Nordin M, Carragee EJ, Hogg-Johnson Sheilah, et. al. Assessment of Neck Pain and Its Associated Disorders: Results of the Bone and Joint Decade 2000-2010 Task Force on Neck Pain and Its Associated Disorders Spine 33(4S): S101-22, 2008.

Ostelo RWJG, Deyo RA, Stratford P, Waddell G, Croft P, Von Korff M, Bouter LM, de Vet HC. Interpreting Change Scores for Pain and Functional Status in Low Back Pain: Towards International Consensus Regarding Minimal Important Change Spine: 33(1): 90-94, 2008.

Paul A, Lewis M, Shadforth MF, Croft PR, Van Der Windt DA, Hay EM. A comparison of four shoulder-specific questionnaires in primary care. Ann Rheum Dis 63 (10): 1293-39, 2004.

Pua YH, Cowan SM, Wrigley TV, Bennell KL. The lower extremity functional scale could be an alternative to the western Ontario and McMaster universities osteoarthritis index physical function scale. J Clin Epidemiol 62 (10): 1103-11, 2009.

Ransford AO, Cairns D, Mooney V. The pain drawing as an aide to the psychologic evaluation of patients with low-back-pain. Spine 1: 127-34, 1976.

Riddle DL, Stratford PW. Use of generic versus region-specific functional status measures on patients with cervical spine disorders. *Phys Ther* 78:951-63, 1998.

Roland M, Morris R. A study of the natural history of back pain. I: Development of a reliable and sensitive measure of disability in low back pain. Spine 1983;8:141-4.

Roland M, Fairbank J. The Roland-Morris Disability Questionnaire and the Oswestry Disability Questionnaire. Spine 2000;25:3115–24.

Salerno DF, Copley-Merriman C, Taylor TN, et. al. A review of functional status measures for workers with upper extremity disorders. Occup Environ Med 59: 664-70, 2002.

Strender LE, Sjoblom A, Sundell K, Ludwig R, Taube A Interexaminer Reliability in Physical Examination of Patients With Low Back Pain Spine 22(7): 814-820, 1997.

Swinkels RA, Oostendorp RA, Bouter LM. Which are the best instruments for measuring disabilities in gait and gait-related activities in patients with rheumatic disorders. Clin Exp Rheumatol 22 (1): 25-33, 2004.

van der Martijn M, Steultjens MPM, Terwee CB, et. al. A systematic review of instruments measuring foot function, foot pain, and foot-related disability in patients with rheumatoid arthritis. Arthritis & Rheumatism 59 (9): 1257-69, 2008.

Ventre J, Schenk RJ Validity of the Duffy-Rath Questionnaire Orthopaedic Practice 17 (1): 22 – 26, 2005.

von Korff M, Jensen MP, Karoly P. Assessing global pain severity by self-report in clinical and health services research. Spine 25 (24):3140–51, 2000.

Wainner RS, Fritz JM, Irrgang JJ, Boninger ML, Delitto A, Allison S. Reliability and Diagnostic Accuracy of the Clinical Examination and Patient Self-Report Measures for Cervical Radiculopathy Spine 28(1): 52-62, 2003.

Wang D, Jones MH, Khair MM, Miniaci A. Patient-reported outcome measures for the knee. J Knee Surg 23 (3): 137-51, 2010.

Zou J, Yang H, Miyazaki M, Wei F, Hong SW, Yoon SH, Morishita Y, Wang JC. Missed Lumbar Disc Herniations Diagnosed With Kinetic Magnetic Resonance Imaging Spine 33(5): E140-44, 2008.

6 BASIC MUSCULOSKELETAL EXAMINATION

The second step in the clinical assessment process is the basic physical examination. This is how you identify the patient's relevant signs and make your diagnosis or prediction of the source of the symptoms; this includes determining the stage (severity) of the disorder. In addition you gain valuable information about how 'irritable' the symptoms are (Rath 1984), and how well the patient is managing/coping with their problem. These findings must be compared to the history and self-reports in the process of coming to your conclusions and developing the most effective initial strategy for each individual patient.

No component of the basic examination is perfunctory and all should be carefully performed. Most importantly, the examination needs to be focused on obtaining the most reliable and relevant clinical information pertinent to each individual patient. This requires the clinician to keep the process as concise and simple as possible (Nelson 1979). The outline of a basic musculoskeletal examination is as follows:

Table 6-1: Outline of the DRS Musculoskeletal Basic Examination
1.   **Observation/Inspection**
1.1 Posture and Body Mechanics
1.2 Visual Inspection: deformity, asymmetry, anomaly, atrophy, disease etc.
1.3 Visual Observation: pattern of movement, non-verbal communication etc.
2.   **Neurologic Screening (PRN)**
2.1 Reflexes (DTR & Cord)
2.2 MMT (motor)
2.3 Sensory
3.   **Motion Assessment (active and passive)**
3.1 Intra-articular
3.2 Extra-articular
3.3 Qualifying tests (e.g. spring testing, CPT etc.)
4.   **Contraction Testing (PRN)**
4.1 Symptom Reproduction Testing
4.2 Strength & Stability Testing
5.   **Palpation (PRN)**
6.   **Auxiliary/Orthopaedic Special Tests (PRN)**

The physical examination is often referred to as the 'objective' component of the assessment; the focus is the identification of signs. According to Taber's Cyclopedic Medical Dictionary; a "sign is an objective evidence of an abnormal nature in the body or its organs.

They are more or less definitive and obvious, and apart from the patient's impressions." (Taber 1963).

These signs can be observed visually, heard, felt and/or recorded. Signs can be measured in degrees, volume, ft. lbs. (parametric), or with numeric rating scale, an ordinal rating scale, a dichotomus rating, etc. (nonparametric). To have meaning the examination procedure has to have a specific intent with an operational definition. Once defined and operationalized it can be evaluated for reliability (intra and inter-rater) and then for validity, provided it is acceptably reliable. A standardization of the physical examination procedures and careful performance leads to a significant improvement in reliability (Strender 1997).

In general, physical examination procedures that have been designed to have an effect on the patient's symptoms are the most reliable and valid (Waddell 1982; Matyas 1985; Nelson 1988; McCombe 1989; Viikari-Juntura 1989; Maher 1994; Sandmark 1995; Donahue 1996; Wainner 2003; Seffinger 2004; Nordin 2008; Vleeming 2008). This is commonsense because symptoms drive patients to treatment, not the asymmetry of a landmark or loss of extensibility of a muscle or an imbalance of proximal strength and motor control. According to Nordin (2008) physical examination procedures that reproduce the symptoms are the gold standard.

1.   **Observation/Inspection** - observation of the patient begins when they enter the waiting room, and continues throughout the time he/she is in your clinic. Gait pattern, biomechanical habits (posture, movement etc.), facial expressions and communication skills are all observed. In the examination room the patient is formally inspected for acute deformity, structural asymmetry, signs of trauma, inflammation, atrophy, trophic changes, rash etc.

2.   **Neurologic screening (PRN)** – assessment of motor and sensory conduction for all appropriate spinal levels. This includes reflex testing (DTR & cord), manual muscle testing (MMT) and sensory evaluation. CNS lesions are identified by a positive Babinsky (i.e. an extensor

response to stroking the sole of the foot), sustained clonus and/or spasticity in response to quick stretch.

When the symptoms are local, behave mechanically and there are no symptoms or signs that could be associated with lesion in the nervous system (central, peripheral or autonomic) these neurologic tests are not required; Bogduk emphasizes this in his textbooks regarding evidence-based assessment and treatment of back and neck pain disorders (2002; 2006). However, these screening procedures only take a minute and it is always best to err on the safe side.

2.1 Reflex testing – the spinal and peripheral nerves are assessed with the DTR tests. The spinal cord and brain are assessed with the Babinsky, Hoffman, clonus and quick stretch tests.

Table 6-2: Grading of the DTR from Loeser (2001). Bigos (1994) suggests that absent, normal, increased or decreased is suitable.	
Grade	**Observation**
0	Absent reflex
Trace	Reflex present only with facilitation (e.g. summation with ValSalva's)
1+ to 3+	Normal range; asymmetry is significant
4+	Pathologically hyperactive; sustained clonus is present.
The most commonly performed deep tendon tests for activity-related spinal disorders.	
DTR	**Level(s) of Test**
Biceps jerk	C5,6 (musculoskeletal nerve)
Triceps jerk	C6,7 (radial nerve)
Wrist jerk	C8, T1 (ulnar nerve)
Knee jerk	L2,3,4 (femoral nerve)
Ankle jerk	S1,2 (tibial nerve)

2.2 Manual Muscle Testing (MMT) – this is testing for radiculopathy or peripheral neuropathy; the weakness should be unequivocal. The muscle grade is usually fair at best and manual resistance easily overcomes the key muscle for the spinal or peripheral nerve involved. A ratchet-like response (i.e. when the power of the muscle alternately increases and decreases during the test) is not possible with radiculopathy or neuropathy.

2.3 Sensory testing – light touch can be used as a quick screen, but pin prick and/or vibration are more reliable tests. Remember that there can be significant individual variability in dermatomes.

2.4 VBI, Cervical Spondylotic Myleopathy, Cauda Equina Compression

– these are three contraindications to physical therapy treatment that clinicians need to be on guard for; the tables below (table 6 -3, 4, 5) review the signs and symptoms for these conditions:

Table 6-3: Signs and symptoms that can be associated with VBI: these are signs and symptoms that can be associated with VBI.	
Symptoms	Signs
Dizziness, disorientation, headache, diplopia, vertigo, tinnitus, blurred vision, feeling cross eyedness, nausea, hallucinosis……….	Dysphagia, dysarthria, nystagmus, drop-attacks, incontinency, Horner's Syndrome, hemiparesis, quadraparesis, ataxia, vomiting, seizure, paralysis of gaze ….

The possibility of vertebral-basilar artery insufficiency (VBI) mimicking or present in conjunction with an ARSD affecting the cervical spine has generated tremendous attention, controversy and concern, especially with manual therapists (APA 1988; Grant 1996; Mitchell 2004; Thiel 2005; Cassidy 2008). This is illustrated in the findings of a meta-analysis examining evidence for efficacy of manual therapy for neck pain (Hurwitz 1996). There was a short-term benefit to both mobilization and manipulation of the neck, but the findings were qualified by a significant possibility for adverse events. Two articles published in the 'Neck Pain Task Force' report for the journal 'Spine' addressed concerns for VBI as the result of chiropractic care (Boyle 2008; Cassidy 2008), finding these events to be rare with no evidence of excess risk from manipulative treatments.

This does not mean there is no risk, as evidenced by the documented incidence of death and serious injury resulting from vertebral artery dissection resulting from sudden manipulation of the neck (Norris 2000; Ernst 2002). In a recent systematic review Ernst (2010) identifies 26 published deaths caused by Chiropractic manipulation, suggests that there are probably more unpublished, and concludes that the risks far out-weigh the benefits of this treatment modality. It is this potential dire consequence that generates the need for hyper diligence. Refer to Chapter 5 for examination procedures and the possible signs and symptoms associated with VBI. When there is any possibility that VBI is present, stop treatment and refer the patient for further medical evaluation.

Regarding the general use of manual therapy, the concepts expressed in McKenzie's paper regarding "Perspectives on Spinal Manipulation" should be followed and I suggest avoiding high velocity upper cervical rotational technique all together for there are so many effective techniques to restore atlanto-axial motion that are gentle and within the patient's ability to stop if the response is inappropriate. It should be noted that in Ernst's recent review there were no known deaths or serious injury caused by physiotherapy manipulation.

Table 6-4: Categories of cervical spondylotic myelopathy (CSM). Taken from Crandal (1966), explained by Hochman (2005).

Category CSM	Signs & Symptoms	Anatomical Basis
The Transverse Lesion	Motor weakness at and below lesion Sensory loss of pain, temp, proprioception, vibration and touch below lesion. Reflexes hyporeflexia at level of lesion, hyperreflexia below lesion.	Degenerative changes damage full diameter of cord leading to damage of the corticospinal and spinothalamic tracts and posterior columns at one of more levels.
The Motor System Syndrome	Motor weakness at level of lesion. Sensory loss of pain and temperature below lesion. Hyporeflexia at level of lesion	Degenerative changes, often by causing vascular compromise (ASA impingement), damage the anterior cord including lower motor neuron nuclei and dessicating pain and temperature fibers at one or more levels.
Central Cord Syndrome	UE > LE weakness below the lesion ("clumsy hands"). Sensory contralateral loss of pain and temperature below the lesion, relative sacral sparing. Hyperreflexia below the lesion.	Degenerative changes cause central cord compression, damaging the corticospinal tracts at one or more levels; medial cervical fibers preferentially damaged over lateral thoracic/lumbar/sacral fibers leading to UE>LE dysfunction.
Brown-Sequard Syndrome	Contralateral weakness below the lesion, ipsilateral weakness at the level. Contralateral sensory loss of pain and temp. below the lesion, ipsilateral loss of proprioception, vibration and touch below the lesion. Ipsilateral hyporeflexia at the level and contralateral hyperreflexia below the lesion.	Degenerative changes damage one side of the cord including the corticospinal and spinothalamic tracts, and posterior columns at one or more levels.
Brachial and Cord Syndrome	Stabbing pain in shoulder and UE, a dull achy feeling in arm. Possible numbness and tingling in hand. May have hyperreflexia below lesion, especially in UE.	Degenerative changes impinging on nerve roots causes brachialgia and mild sensory changes; may have hyperreflexia from early corticospinal tract involvement.

Cord compression occurring as a result of spondylosis and/or a HNP is most likely to occur in the cervical spine, but can also occur in the thoracic region. The patient's history will suggest the presence of myelopathy but the results of the neurologic examination and diagnostic tests ultimately make the diagnosis. Regarding incidence and prevalence, cervical spondylotic radiculomyelopathy is significantly greater than cauda equina syndrome, but the indication for surgery and expected outcome is not as clear (Morio 2000; Fouyas 2002; Ishida 2002; Kadanka 2000, 2002; Yamazaki 2003; Ogawa 2006; Rhee 2009; Cunningham 2010). Factors affecting surgical outcome include severity of neurologic damage, duration of the condition (time from onset to surgery), age of the patient, the transverse diameter of the spinal cord at the level of the lesion and more.

Table 6-5: Signs and symptoms associated with Cauda Equina Compression	
Symptoms	Signs
Saddle numbness is the primary symptom report; can be associated with report of progressive weakness in legs and/or bilateral radicular pain.	Saddle anesthesia, loss of anal sphincter tone and reflex, loss of bowel (incontinence) or bladder control (incontinence or inability to initiate urination), male impotence, progressive multi-level radiculopathy.

Early recognition of the cauda equina syndrome is critical because this is a surgical emergency to prevent permanent neurologic damage. Fortunately the incidence is low, calculated to be 3.4/1.5 per million annually (Podnar 2007) and the surgical outcome is usually good with quick recognition (Kostuik 1986; Shapiro 2000). The symptoms often include bilateral sciatica, but not always. The neurologic disturbance can affect bladder and/or bowel control, but progressive deficits affecting multiple root levels is also evidence and should prompt immediate medical evaluation. Although a large centrally located HNP is the most common cause of a cauda equina syndrome it can also be a result of spinal stenosis, primary or metastatic tumor, infectious diseases, A-V malformation, hemorrhage or iatrogenic causes (Todd 2009).

3. Motion Assessment – this includes the assessment of intra-articular (i.e. a joint dysfunction) and extra-articular (i.e. outside of the joint; multi-joint muscle extensibility, neural tension testing etc.) and the relevance of any findings to 'the' patient's symptoms or activity-related dysfunction. This is a critical part of the examination process and frequently these tests pinpoint the source of the patient's symptoms and direct the initial treatment plan. Consequently the remaining procedures in the basic examination are only performed when needed.

Note: It is very important to explain to the patient that you are looking to determine if any of the tests affect the symptoms identified in the history to be relevant (i.e. 'the' symptoms). Most of the examination tests and treatment procedures cause a normal symptom response (e.g. strain, pressure, stretch etc.), so it is important not to confuse this response as being relevant to the pain generator. The relevance of a loss of motion is determined by an increase or decrease of the relevant symptoms; we call this **'directly relevant'** *(see below). This applies to the other basic examination tests and procedures, is a fundamental premise in the Duffy-Rath System©, and a critical component to reliability and validity of physical examination procedures.*

Ultimately there are three questions to be answered after completing the motion assessment:

One: Is there any loss of motion, and if so in what directions?
Two: If so, was the loss relevant to 'the' symptoms?
Three: If relevant, is the loss inside and/or outside the joint(s)?

In the DRS there are 2 categories of relevant signs; 1) directly relevant and 2) indirectly relevant. This mostly applies when the examiner identifies a loss of motion and/or abnormal muscle contraction responses. The following defines these two categories of relevance as they relate to the motion loss assessment:

Directly relevant – the movements identified to be limited reproduce (or diminish) 'the' symptoms, i.e. they directly affect the symptoms.

Indirectly relevant – the limited movements do not reproduce 'the' symptoms but they do have an adverse effect on biomechanical control during activity and function (e.g. loss of hip flexor extensibility is not the source of symptoms with a relevant spondylolisthesis but when you have established that controlling lumbar extension during standing activities reduces 'the' pain then improving hip flexor extensibility can increase the patient's biomechanical control over their problem during upright activities).

Differentiating the source of relevant motion loss "Inside &/or Outside of the Joints"

Determining the source of the relevant motion loss is an essential goal of the physical examination. This requires discipline with attention to controlling the mechanical and physiological effects of the testing procedures.

Step 1: the first goal of the examination is to determine whether or not there is a loss of normal joint motion - this requires a definition. In the DRS we define normal joint motion as; the ability to move the joint passively from mid-range to end range without pain or any abnormal symptom response, and accept overpressure at end range with a normal mechanical and symptomatic response. And this is repeatable in all directions the joints under investigation are designed to move and there are no adverse effect on opposite movements.

Passive range of motion (PROM) is the most reliable way to assess for joint motion loss because it eliminates contraction of the muscles, controls the kinematics and is required for testing overpressure. In many cases, particularly when screening for motion loss you can have the patient actively move to end range and then add passive overpressure. Patients that cannot relax enough to allow you to move them through their available ROM present a particular challenge to coming to a conclusion about the source of 'the' symptoms and they require special attention and consideration (this is covered later).

The next consideration in assessing joint motion is to make sure that the multi-joint muscles and connective tissues that could mechanically interfere with the available ROM are put on slack so that they do not affect the results of the test.

The comparison of available ROM and effect on symptom reproduction when motion is tested with and without external tension is critical to determining the source(s) of the symptoms. Examples include: testing lumbar flexion sitting verses standing; cervical side-bending with and without the shoulder and upper limb tension structures supported and on slack; wrist extension with elbows bent and forearms neutral verses with elbow extended and forearm fully supinated; shoulder external rotation at 0 degrees verses 90 degrees abduction etc.

Another qualifying test is to apply manual overpressure to the joint at end range; in the spine this is called a 'spring test'. When this is performed with the external structures off tension and the symptoms are reproduced the source of the symptoms is the joint or some structure that is being pinched within the joint.

Step 1 Conclusions - at the completion of step 1 you should have identified or ruled-out the joint as the source, or a source of the patient's symptoms. The problem is clearly in the joint complex when passive motion is unequivocally limited and reproduces 'the' pain when tested. Compare to the other side when available.

The jury is still out when there is no loss of motion but there is a reproduction of 'the' pain at end range and/or with over pressure. This could indicate stretching or compression of an external joint structure, or initial evidence for joint instability. To sort this out you need to:

1. Make certain you removed external tension – if this eliminates the symptom response then you need to specifically test the external structures to determine source (i.e. specific muscle length tests, contraction testing, neural tension testing etc.). **Go to step 2.**

2. Test and assess joint stability – manual overpressure is the essence of ligament integrity testing (e.g. varus and valgus stress testing etc.) and problems with joint instability are exposed under load (e.g. in weight bearing, while exerting force especially when at end range etc.). When there is evidence for reproduction of symptoms with PROM, and both abnormal play with end range overpressure and intolerance to loading during function a case for joint instability has been established.

Certain joints are more vulnerable to this than others; e.g. gleno-humeral joint, wrist joint, 1st CMC, lumbo-sacral and upper cervical spine.

Step 2 - the second goal of the examination is to determine if there is any relevant loss of external, multi-joint extensibility.

This is critical to establishing the source of the symptoms when PROM of the joint is found to be full with no symptom reproduction. When the joint has been implicated, this identifies if there is more than one source of the symptoms and/or if a loss of external extensibility is a predisposing factor or an indirectly relevant sign.

Step 2 involves testing the available ROM and effect on symptoms when specific multi-joint muscles or connective tissues are placed on tension; e.g. ability to move and response of symptoms when attempting to extend the lumbar spine with hip flexors or rectus femoris on tension, or cervical side-bend away when an upper limb tension test is performed; or extend the wrist when the elbow is extended and forearm fully supinated etc.

When the ROM is abnormally limited and 'the' symptoms are reproduced when external tension is present and then the motion is full and no symptoms reproduced when tension is removed the source is external to the joint(s).

Many of the biomechanical problems associated with loss of multi-joint extensibility have the possibility of being a muscular, peripheral nerve or nerve root dysfunction. A classic example would be a loss of motion and reproduction of symptoms with SLR occurs with a hamstring injury, a lower lumbar/upper sacral nerve root disorder or a peripheral entrapment neuropathy of the sciatic nerve.

The key to differentiating these sources is a combination of clarifying the patient history, remaining objective about the signs and symptoms of peripheral neuropathy and radicular pain or radiculopathy, and performing qualifying tests that help to localize the source.

Nerve root – a nerve root disorder is often a progression of a back or neck problem, so look for the symptoms at onset to be in those regions or at least a previous history. Look for back or neck motions to affect the symptoms; the symptoms should follow a root distribution, and most importantly know your definitions; radicular pain (IASP): "Pain perceived as arising in a limb or the trunk wall caused by ectopic activation of nociceptive afferent fibers in a spinal nerve or its roots or other neuropathic mechanisms. The pain is lancinating in quality and travels along a narrow band. It may be episodic, recurrent, or paroxysmal according to the causative lesion or any superimposed aggravating factors." The root is identified when root tension tests, especially when adding dural tension (e.g. cervical flexion, ankle DF etc.) reproduce the symptoms. When the radicular pain includes a radiculopathy, then the examination identifies specific weakness and/or loss of cutaneous sensibility specific to a root level.

Peripheral Nerve – a peripheral nerve disorder is associated with very specific signs and symptoms related to dysfunction of the nerve involved. You need to know whether or not that particular nerve has a sensory and/or a motor supply. The patient's symptoms (neuralgia) need to be consistent with neuropathy (i.e. in distribution of the nerve, reported as paresthesia, analgesia, hyperalgesia, causalgia) and the examination should then identify the specific loss of cutaneous sensibility and/or muscle weakness in distribution. In addition there can be positive neural tension testing – but this would be secondary to the previous signs and symptoms identified.

Muscular Injury – direct injuries to the muscles either involve a traumatic event, an incident (A or B) involving force exertion or a delayed (usually next day) response to an increase in physical demands and/or exertions to which the patient is not accustomed. In the last case there is no one incident or event; plus there is always the possibility of a completely insidious onset.

The symptoms are local to the injury site ± referred, and contraction testing clearly and consistently reproduces 'the' symptoms. There is a conspicuous absence of signs and symptoms that differentiate a nerve root or peripheral nerve disorder.

When the joint has been ruled-out or is not the sole source, and a nerve root and/or peripheral nerve has also been eliminated you must proceed to the next step in the basic examination; contraction testing.

The Neural tension tests

There are 2 general groups of neural tension tests; those that focus on assessing for adverse nerve root tension and those that focus on the peripheral nerves. There are numerous causes for adverse neural tension. Each test should be performed carefully and meticulously, going only to the point where symptoms are reproduced. Since these tests also affect multi-joint muscles refer to the previous section on how to differentiate muscle, root and peripheral nerve. The following are the most commonly employed neural tension tests:

SLR (straight leg raise) – roots of sacral plexus and sciatic nerve

FNS (femoral nerve stretch) – roots of lumbar plexus and femoral nerve

ULTT (upper limb tension test) – roots, trunks and cords of brachial plexus - modifications to the basic test for the radial, ulnar and median nerves

4. Contraction Testing

This involves an assessment of either the effect of contraction of the muscles in reproducing 'the' symptoms (direct relevance) or the identification of weakness and/or imbalance that could be indirectly relevant. There are 2 groups of contraction testing procedures: 1) specific, joint neutral manual muscle testing procedures when the muscle/tendon is suspected of being the source, and 2) classic muscle and strength testing procedures when assessing for weakness, imbalance and/or dynamic stabilization.

Joint Neutral Contraction Testing – this is an isometric contraction test with the joint placed in a neutral (mid-range) position in attempt to control stress and strain to the capsule, ligaments and intra-articular structures. The patient is provided an explanation of the test and the resistance is slowly and progressively applied until either 'the' symptoms are reproduced (stop at the point where the symptoms start) or the muscle breaks indicating maximal contraction was achieved.

A positive test is a reproduction of 'the' pain. However, confirming that the source of the symptoms is in the muscle/tendon is not that simple. You need to see a pattern of response that is consistent with the mechanical function of the specific muscle/tendon unit. When the source of the symptoms is the muscle/tendon the response to contraction testing should be consistent. Although the intent is not to test the muscle beyond the point of symptom reproduction, the patient's response should be: the greater the intensity of the contraction the greater the intensity of the pain report. Palpation is then utilized to locate the exact site of the lesion when within reach.

Therefore the positive contraction test is <u>not</u> identifying the muscle/tendon as the source when: 1) the greatest symptom response is upon the release of the contraction, 2) repositioning the joint(s) eliminates the pain response, 3) as the intensity of contraction increases the symptom response does not, 4) the symptoms are reproduced by opposite movements (e.g. resisting abduction and adduction; internal and external rotation, etc.) or 3) stabilizing the joint eliminates the symptom response. These responses indicate the symptoms are emanating from a bursa and/or involve joint instability – or possibly you are testing the wrong region (e.g. shoulder contraction testing can reproduce pain coming from a mechanical lower neck disorder).

Classic Muscle & Strength Testing – this is performed with the intent of looking for evidence of weakness, imbalance or lack of biomechanical control; all of which could be predisposing (indirectly relevant) factors.

These tests are not required at most initial assessment sessions because the start of treatment usually involves controlling the relevant symptoms; they are certainly not indicated S/P trauma or with acute, irritable conditions. However, with chronic conditions and/or when there is evidence of instability this information may be very important to developing an initial strategy and consequently a component of the initial assessment.

The specific tests performed are covered in each of the three region workshops (i.e. the back, neck and limbs). In the DRS these tests include traditional MMT grading of strength, a DRS grading system for trunk strength, standardized testing (e.g. grip and pinch strength measures etc.) and functional testing (e.g. lift, carry, climb capacity etc.). Comparison to normative data is encouraged when available, and most importantly assessment in relation to the physical demands of the individual patient's lifestyle.

A commitment to ongoing, strategic strength and conditioning is a core element of the DRS and is essential to maintaining activity tolerance and preventing MSD for a lifetime.

Palpation

Manual palpation skills are very important to confirming certain diagnoses and/or directing treatment to the correct location for certain disorders. However, palpation alone is not a reliable diagnostic tool and can lead to a misdirection of treatment, resulting in inefficient, ineffective and/or misinterpreted outcomes. A skilled musculoskeletal clinician can accurately identify all the relevant anatomical landmarks, structural locations, articular levels and components of the spine and extremities. Therefore, in the DRS we encourage clinicians to become highly adept at musculoskeletal palpation techniques, but then to follow application guidelines:

- Palpation has value as an adjunct diagnostic, or as a therapeutic tool only when the structure or tissue is within palpation's reach.
- Only use palpation to confirm a musculoskeletal diagnosis after you have deduced the most likely source of the symptoms by correlating history, motion loss, contraction, ± auxiliary testing.

- When using palpation to locate the site of the lesion or disorder do not confuse normal tenderness with a reproduction of 'the' pain; keep in mind the definition of chronic widespread pain (and other causes of hyperesthesia). Compare to opposite limb or other unaffected spinal regions.

5. Auxiliary tests (Orthopaedic special tests)

Auxiliary or orthopaedic special tests (OST) are abundant in musculoskeletal healthcare. The practice of assigning one's name to a procedure alleged or proven to establish a MSD has been common for centuries; e.g. Thomas Test for the hip, Finklestein's for the thumb, Tinel's, Jobe's, Hawkins etc.

These special tests are purported to establish or refute a diagnosis so the most appropriate treatment plan can be developed – a classic biomedical approach to treatment. However, the number of OST that have accumulated is staggering and many have the same problem as diagnostic imaging; sensitive but not specific.

In the DRS we use OST sparingly, and only those that are based upon reproducing 'the' symptoms and/or proven high diagnostic accuracy and strong likelihood ratios (positive and negative).

References Chapter 6

Australian Physiotherapy Association (APA). Protocol for premanipulative testing of the cervical spine. Australian Journal of Physiotherapy 34:97–100, 1988.

Bigos S, Bowyer O, Braen G, et. al. Acute Low back Problems in Adults. Clinical Practice Guidelines No. 14. AHCPR Publication No. 95-0642. Rockville, MD: Agency for health Care Policy and Research, Public Health Service, US Department of Health and Human Services. December 1994.

Bogduk N, Munro RR. Experimental low back pain, referred pain and muscle spasm. Journal of Anatomy 1979;128:661.

Bogduk N, Govind J. Medical Management of Acute Lumbar Radicular Pain: An Evidence-based Approach. New South Wales, Newcastle Bone and Joint Institute, 1999a.

Bogduk N, Govind J. Medical Management of Acute Cervical Radicular Pain: An Evidence-based Approach. New South Wales, Newcastle Bone and Joint Institute, 1999b.

Bogduk N, McGuirk B. Pain Research and Clinical Management; Vol. 13: Medical Management of Acute and Chronic Low Back Pain. An Evidence-based Approach. Elsevier, Amsterdam, 2002.

Bogduk N, McGuirk B. Pain Research and Clinical Management: Pain Research and Clinical Management of Acute and Chronic Neck Pain. An Evidence-based Approach. Edinburgh, Elsevier, 2006.

Boyle E, Cote P, Grier AR, Cassidy JD. Examining Vertebrobasilar Artery Stroke in Two Canadian Provinces. Spine 33 (4S): S170-75, 2008.
Brieg A. Marions O. Biomechanics of the lumbosacral nerve roots. Acta Radiologica (Diagnosis) 1: 1141- 60, 1963.

Brieg A Adverse Mechanical Tension in the Central Nervous System. New York, John Wiley & Sons 1978.

Breig A, Troup JD. Biomechanical considerations in the straight-leg-raising test: cadaveric and clinical studies of the effects of medial hip rotation. Spine 4 (3): 242-5, 1979.

Butler DS. Mobilisation of the Nervous System. Melbourne, Churchill Livingstone, 1991.

Cassidy JD, Boyle E, Cote P, He Y, Hogg-Johnson S, Silver FL, Bondy SJ. Risk of Vertebrobasilar Stroke and Chiropractic Care Results of a Population-Based Case-Control and Case-Crossover Study. Spine 33 (4S): S176-83, 2008.

Coman WB. Dizziness related to ENT conditions. In: Grieve G P (ed) Modern manual therapy of the vertebral column. Churchill Livingstone, Edinburgh, pp. 303-314, 1986.

Crandall PH, Batzdorf U. Cervical spondylotic myelopathy. J Neurosurg 25: 57-66, 1966.

Cunningham MR, Hershman S, Bendo J. Systematic review of cohort studies comparing surgical treatment for cervical sponylotic myelopathy. Spine 35 (5): 537-43, 2010.

Cyriax J: Mechanism of Symptoms: Dural pain. Lancet 29 (April):919-921,1978.

Cyriax J: Textbook of Orthopaedic Medicine: Vol I. Diagnosis of Soft Tissue Lesions, 8th Edition. London, Bailliere Tindall, 1982.

Donahue MS, Riddle DL, Sullivan MS. Intertester reliability of a modified version of McKenzie's lateral shift assessments obtained on patients with low back pain Phys Ther 76 (7): 706-716, 1996.

Dvořák J Neurophysiologic tests in diagnosis of nerve root compression caused by disc herniation. Spine 21(24S): 39S-44S, 1996.

Dyck P. The femoral nerve traction test with lumbar disc protrusions. Surg Neurol 6:163-7, 1976.

Elvy RL Treatment of arm pain associated with abnormal brachial plexus tension. Australian J Physiotherapy 32(4): 225-30, 1986.

Elvy RL. The investigation of arm pain. In Gieve GP, Ed. Modern Manual Therapy of the Vertebral Column. Churchill Livingstone, Edinburgh, 1986: pp. 530-35.

Ernst E. Manipulation of the cervical spine: a systematic review of case reports of serious adverse events, 1995-2001. Med J Aust 176: 376-80, 2002.

Ernst E. Deaths after chiropractic: a review of published cases. Int J Clin Pract 64 (10): 1162-65, 2010.

Estridge MN, Rouhe SA, Johnson NG. The femoral stretching test: A valuable sign in diagnosing upper lumbar disc herniation. J Neurosurg 57:813-17, 1982.

Fouyas IP, Statham PFX, Sandercock PAG. Cochrane review on the role of surgery in cervical spondylotic radiculomyeopathy. Spine 27 (7): 736-47, 2002.

Gonnella C, Paris SV, Kutner M: Reliability in Evaluating Passive Intervertebral Motion. Phy Ther 62: 436-444, 1982.

Grant R. Vertebral artery testing – the Australian Physiotherapy Association protocol after 6 years. Manual Therapy 1 (3): 149-53, 1996.

Hochman M, Tuli S. Cervical spondylotic myelopathy: a review. The Internet Journal of Neurology. 2005; Volume 4, Number 1.

Hurwitz EL, Aker PD, Adams AH, et. al. Manipulation and mobilization of the cervical spine. A systematic review of the literature. Spine 21 (15): 1746-59, 1996.

Ishida, Y, Tominaga, T. Predictors of neurologic recovery in acute central cervical cord injury with only upper extremity impairment. Spine 27 (15): 1652 – 57, 2002.

Jull G, Zito G, Trott P, Potter H, Shirley D, Richardson C. Inter-examiner reliability to detect painful upper cervical joint dysfunction. Australian Physiother J 43 (2): 125-129, 1997.

Kadanka, Z, Bednarik, J, Vohanka, S, et al. Conservative treatment versus surgery in spondylotic cervical myelopathy: a prospective randomised study. Eur Spine Journal 9(6):538 – 44, 2000.

Kadanka Z, Mares M, Bednanik J, et. al. Approaches to spondylotic cervical myelopathy: conservative versus surgical results in a 3-year follow-up study. Spine 27 (20): 2205 – 10, 2002.

Kendall FP, McCreary EK, Provance PG. Muscles Testing and Function, 4th E: with posture and pain. Williams & Wilkins, Baltimore, 1993.

Kostuik JP, Harrington I, Alexander D, et al. Cauda equina syndrome and lumbar disc herniation. JBJS 68A (3): 386-91, 1986.

Lasègue C. Considérations sur la sciatique. Arch Gen Med (Paris). 2: 558-80, 1984.

Laslett M, William M: The reliability of selected pain provocation tests for sacroiliac joint pathology. Spine 19 (11): 1243-1249, 1994.

Loeser JG. Medical evaluation of the patient with pain. In. Loeser JD (Editor). Bonica's Management of Pain, 3rd edition. Philadelphia, Lippincott Williams & Wilkins, 2001; 267-78.

Maher C, Adams R. Reliability of pain and stiffness assessments in clinical manual lumbar spine examination. Physical Therapy 74(9): 801-809, 1994.

Matyas TA and Bach TM: The Reliability of Selected Techniques in Clinical Arthrometrics. Australian J Physiother 31 (5): 175-195, 1985.

McCombe PF, Fairbank JCT, Cockersole BC, et al: Reproducibility of Physical Signs in Low-Back Pain. Spine 14 (9): 908-918, 1989.

Mitchell J, Keene D, Dyson C, Harvey L, Pruvey C, Phillips R. Is cervical spine rotation, as used in the standard vertebrobasilar insufficiency test, associated with a measureable change in intracranial vertebral artery blood flow? Manual Therapy 9(4): 220-27, 2004.

Morio, Y, Teshima, R, Nagashima, H, et al. Correlation between operative outcomes of cervical compression myelopathy and MRI of the spinal cord. Spine 26 (11):1238 - 45, 2001.

Nelson MA, Allen MB, Clamp SE, et al: Reliability and Reproducibility of Clinical Findings in Low-Back Pain. Spine 4 (2): 97-101, 1979.

Nordin M, Carragee EJ, Hogg-Johnson Sheilah, et. al. Assessment of Neck Pain and Its Associated Disorders: Results of the Bone and Joint Decade 2000-2010 Task Force on Neck Pain and Its Associated Disorders Spine 33(4S): S101-22, 2008.

Norris JW, Beletsky V, Nadareishvili ZG. Sudden neck movement and cervical artery dissection. The Canadian Stroke Consortium. CMAJ 163: 38-40, 2000.

Ogawa, Y, Chiba, K, Matsumoto, M, et al. Postoperative factors affecting neurological recovery after surgery for cervical spondylotic myelopathy. J Neurosurg Spine 5:483 – 87, 2006.

Podnar S. Epidemiology of cauda and conus medullaris equina lesions. Muscle & Nerve 35 (4): 529-31, 2007.

Rath W. Cervical Traction, a Clinical Perspective. Orthopaedic Review 13 (8): 29-48, 1984.

Rhee JM, Heflin JA, Hamasaki T, Freedman B. Prevalence of Physical Signs in Cervical Myelopathy A Prospective, Controlled Study. Spine 34 (9): 890-95, 2009.

Rubinstein SM, Pool JJM, van Tulder MW, Riphagen II, de Vet HCW. A systematic review of the diagnostic accuracy of provocative tests of the neck for diagnosing cervical radiculopathy. Eur Spine J 16: 307-19, 2007.

Sandmark H, Nisell R. Validity of five common manual neck pain provoking tests. Scand J Rehabil Med 27: 131-6, 1995.

Seffinger MA, Najm WI, Mishra SI, et. al. Reliability of spinal palpation for diagnosis of back and neck pain: a systematic review of the literature. Spine 29 (19): E413-25, 2004.

Shapiro S. Medical realities of cauda equina syndrome secondary to lumbar disc herniation. Spine 25 (3): 348 – 52, 2000.

Sommerfeld P, Kaider A, Klein P. Inter- and intraexaminer reliability in palpation of the "primary respiratory mechanism" within the "cranial concept". Manual Therapy 9 (1): 22–29, 2004.

Spitzer WO, LeBlanc FE, Dupuis M, et al: Scientific Approach to the Assessment and Management of Activity-related Spinal Disorders. Spine 12 (7S) 1987.

Spitzer WO, Skovron ML, Salmi LR, Cassidy JD, et al. Scientific monograph of the Quebec task force on whiplash-associated disorders: redefining 'whiplash' and its management. Spine 20 (8S), 1995.

Strender LE, Sjoblom A, Sundell K, Ludwig R, Taube A Interexaminer Reliability in Physical Examination of Patients With Low Back Pain Spine 22(7): 814-820, 1997.

Taber CW. Taber's Cyclopedic Medical Dictionary, 9th Ed. Philadelphia, FA Davis, 1963.

Thiel H, Rix G. Is it time to stop functional pre-manipulation testing of the cervical spine? Manual Therapy 10 (2): 154-58, 2005.

Todd NV. An algorithm for suspected cauda equina syndrome. Ann R Coll Surg Engl 19 (4): 358-9, 2009.

Viikari-Juntura E, Porras M, Laasonen EM. Validity of clinical tests in the diagnosis of root compression in cervical disc disease. Spine 14 (3): 253-7, 1989.

Vleeming A, Albert HB, Östgaard HC, Sturesson B, Stuge B. European guidelines for the diagnosis and treatment of pelvic girdle pain. Eur Spine J DOI 10.1007/s00586-008-0602-4, Springer-Verlag 2008.

Waddell G, Main CJ, Morris EW, Venner RM, Rae P, Sharmy SH, Galloway H. Normality and reliability in the clinical assessment of backache. Br Med J 284: 1519-23, 1982.

Wainner RS, Fritz JM, Irrgang JJ, Boninger ML, DeLitto A, Allison S. Reliability and diagnostic accuracy of the clinical examination and patient self-report measures for cervical radiculopathy. Spine 28(1): 52-62, 2003.

Yamazaki, T, Yanaka, K, Sato, H, et al. Cervical spondylotic myelopathy: surgical results and factors affecting outcome with special reference to age differences. Neurosurgery 52 (1):122 – 26, 2003.

7 EXAMINATION CONCLUSIONS

The purpose of the history-taking and the physical examination process is to provide the clinician with enough information to establish a preliminary conclusion and initiate an appropriate treatment plan. These conclusions include establishing a diagnosis whenever possible or identifying sub-groups when the disorder is nonspecific. This is addressed for each musculoskeletal region in the workshop series. However, it is well established that regardless of diagnosis a biopsychosocial model of care is needed if the goal is to prevent disability and have a long-term (positive) impact.

Our system guides the treatment decision process by categorizing the severity of the patient's condition (i.e. stage of the disorder), identifying the clinical characteristics of their symptoms and signs (i.e. 3x3 determination of clinical state), the impact of other factors, and ultimately by the response of the patient to the initial assessment and treatment process. The initial assessment process also screens for the presence of contraindications or cautions to physical therapy treatments (covered in a separate chapter).

Stage of the Musculoskeletal Disorders

We developed the 3-stages concept in 1984 to explain to patients the progression and remission of the symptoms and signs of cumulative strain disorders. The intent was to relate the concept to their specific case so they could understand how to gain control and take an active role in recovery. As a result they learned the skills required to prevent recurrence, and maintain physical performance capabilities. This was intricately connected to our philosophical position that all cumulative strain disorders are inherently preventable provided the root causes are addressed at or before the warning signal stage – see table 7-1 below.

This is also a tool that helps clinicians recognize the severity of the MSD which will ultimately affect expectations, reliability of diagnoses, resource utilization, the initial verses eventual treatment strategy, choice of specific treatment procedures, and the need for specialist referral.

Table 7-1: The Duffy-Rath 3-Stages of Musculoskeletal Disorders: All cumulative disorders pass through stage one and are inherently preventable, representing the opportunity for primary prevention. Stage 2 provides the opportunity for secondary prevention and stage three is either secondary or tertiary.		
Stage 1 – Warning Signals	Stage 2 – Nonspecific Disorder	Stage 3 – Structural Pathology
Stable intermittent symptoms produced as a result of fatigue of passive and/or dynamic connective tissues. No consequence to symptom production and no <u>directly relevant</u> signs.	Progression of symptoms to unstable intermittent or constant. Emergence of directly relevant signs. At least some degree of interference with normal levels of physical activity – rapidly reversible with early intervention that addresses root issues ± natural history.	Signs and symptoms unequivocally associated with a pathoanatomical diagnosis (e.g. radiculopathy, tendon rupture, joint instability, advanced OA etc.) – slowly recovers to potential, potentially irreversible in some cases with the need to adjust functional goals accordingly.

As a general rule you should start your treatment programs conservatively (e.g. anti-inflammatory or posture-ergonomic strategy) with all stage 3 disorders and S/P trauma (see separate chapter for more information) – even if you feel there is a possibility for rapid response.

3 X 3 Clinical State of the Patient's MSD

The clinical state of the patient refers to the stability of the patient's symptoms and signs. We developed this concept as a general guide for how conservatively or how aggressively you should start a treatment program for an MSD (Rath 1984). The top row of the table below indicates the need for the most conservative start; the bottom (third) row suggests a more aggressive approach should be well tolerated. We refer to the degree of irritability throughout the workshop series as an important assessment factor in your clinical decision making process – see table 7-2 below.

Other Factors

The presence of comorbidities (i.e. coexisting diseases, disorders or confounding factors) should influence your conclusions and choice of the initial treatment strategy – ultimately this affects the setting of functional goals and overall expectations for response. This includes assessment of the patient's response to their musculoskeletal problem – when significantly distressed, poor coping skills or other psychosocial and/or fear-avoidance behaviors predominate - your choice of the best treatment plan has to be affected.

Table 7-2: 3 x 3 Determination of clinical state (Rath 1984) – this was proposed as a general guideline for starting a treatment stage; i.e. very conservative or aggressively.

Stage of Healing (S/P trauma when applicable)	State of the Joint(s) (Response to motion assessment)	Degree of Irritability (Response after exam or treatment procedure)
Exudative phase: 3 – 10 days	Acute: pain prior to reaching end range	Maximal: minimal provocation reproduces a lasting increase of symptoms.
Fibroblastic phase: up to 25 days following resolution of exudative phase	Subacute: pain upon reaching end range	Moderate: a moderate amount of provocation reproduces symptoms that slowly subside.
Remodeling phase: indefinite time period depending upon severity of tissue damage.	Chronic: pain only upon applying overpressure at end range	Minimal: significant amount of provocation reproduces minimal symptoms that quickly subside.

The Duffy-Rath Response Groups

As previously stated, how we initiate a treatment plan is based on the patient's stage of disorder, their clinical state, and how they responded to history, physical examination and any trial treatment procedures. Over the years we have identified 5 general categories that predict how quickly we expect the patient to respond, how conservatively we need to start and what clinical paradigm to use to achieve functional and long-term goals. We call these categories our 'response-based conclusions' and they are directly linked to DRS treatment strategies (covered in detail in the next chapter). The 5 categories or response groups are; rapid responder, cumulative responder, adverse responder, non-mechanical responder and other.

Rapid response group – the examination and the first treatment has demonstrated the ability to consistently control the relevant symptoms and signs (RSSx) with biomechanical instruction and/or manual/mechanical procedures. These improvements are consistent, comprehensive and functionally stable; i.e. remain better when challenged. A rapid response is commonly found with early interventions for minor MSD; i.e. stage 1 or stage 2 disorders with a consistent mechanical pattern of response. Rarely does a stage 3 disorder rapidly respond, even when the symptoms can be fully controlled either the signs do not quickly resolve and/or the patient is unable to return to full activity and functional tolerance right away. Musculoskeletal self-efficacy is encouraged when the patient actively participates in their recovery and experiences how they can control their RSSx – what we refer to as experiencing the positive 'cause and effect' of their actions.

Cumulative response group – the RSSx cannot be fully controlled and/or does not result in a quick or complete restoration of the patient's lost activity tolerances. In other words, improvements are partial and require a progression of treatment procedures that gradually result in a complete or 'to potential' recovery of activity tolerance. A cumulative response is expected with many chronic disorders or major MSD (e.g. ruptured disc, RCT etc.) that are in the rehabilitation phase of management; i.e. chronic stage 2 or stage 3 disorders. This gives ample opportunity to build musculoskeletal self-efficacy provided the message is consistent throughout the progression of treatment.

Adverse response group – the RSSx are unstable, easily provoked with lasting consequences and/or this is a major MSD in the early (acute) stages of management. This conclusion prompts a conservative start to treatment that is focused on control of symptoms and aggravating factors; the relevant signs are not directly addressed. This is a good initial strategy when you are not confident about how the patient will respond to treatment and/or there is evidence that they could easily flare. When a patient has constant or unstable intermittent pain that is severe and/or can easily flare you immediately gain their confidence when you are able to consistently control the symptoms – we use patient positioning and mid-range biomechanical procedures to accomplish this, sometimes in conjunction with medically prescribed medications and/or injections.

Non-mechanical response group – in this group there are disproportionately severe symptoms with a lack of corresponding signs; or there are signs that are inconsistent, labile and/or cannot explain or predict symptom behavior. This is found with chronic widespread pain and/or with patients with predominant fear-avoidance behaviors; what Waddell called 'non-organic' presentations. This group can respond well provided the treatment paradigm is adjusted appropriately – usually the improvements are cumulative and consistent with remodeling. Building patient self-efficacy can be a challenge, always requiring consistent reinforcement and positive messaging.

Other - this group captures those patients that do not fit into the main categories; either they do not have an activity-related MSD, they did not come to you for treatment (e.g. consultation, FCE etc.), or they just don't fit into the main groupings.

The Response-based Conclusion Should Match the Treatment Strategy (table 7-3) - your clinical conclusions guide your choice of treatment strategy in the DRS. Over many years of treatment and prevention experience we have identified six general treatment strategies to successfully manage a large cross-section of patients with MSD. These six strategies correlate to the response group conclusions, as follows (to be covered in detail in Chapter 11):

Table 7-3: The four response groups correspond to one of six DRS treatment strategies.	
Response-based Conclusion	**Treatment Strategy**
Rapid response	Postural-ergonomic
Rapid response	Reduction
Adverse response	Anti-inflammatory
Cumulative response	Remodeling
Cumulative response	Stabilization

DRS Response Group & Treatment Strategy Flow-Sheet (Figure 7-1)

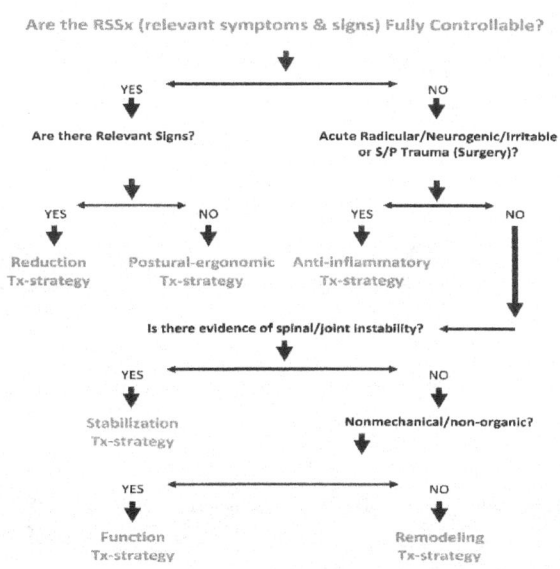

This flowchart presumes that patients with contraindications ('red flags') and medical conditions have been ruled-out.

Expectations for Response to Treatment

Our experience and expectation is that most patients with an MSD seen for treatment will respond predictably and rapidly; however this is significantly affected by how quickly you intervene after onset (i.e. acute and subacute tend to respond more quickly than chronic), the stage of the disorder (e.g. radiculopathy responds more slowly than nonspecific back and neck pain), the activity status of the patient at the time of the initial evaluation (i.e. active responds more quickly than idle). Even chronic disorders can respond rapidly provided the symptoms and signs behave mechanically and the patient has remained reasonably active, fit and conditioned. Individual expectations of the therapist and the patient are becoming recognized as a relevant factor that influences outcomes (Bialosky 2012).

Regardless of how rapidly the patient responds you need to assess how well they are prepared for the long-term management of their problem and physical performance capabilities. In fact patients that recover very quickly and easily may not appreciate the need for change in their habits and behaviors because the problem does not appear significant and their experience is that they can fix it if it returns. This is most likely if their treatment was passive and the therapist did not address the long-term issue directly.

Our overall expectation is that 90 – 95% of the patients with an MSD that come to your service should respond to your treatment. How many respond rapidly versus slowly differs with the practitioner, treatment approach and the population of patients; along with many other factors.

Below are the results of a consecutive case series investigation involving 7 physical therapists who completed DRS certification (tables 7-4,5,6,7). These results are similar to ongoing data from our clinics over the past 25 years – this can be used as a general guide for expectations of response using a DRS-like approach to the treatment of ARMSD. The first table presents outcomes; the second and third table present the change in pain and self-rated disability scores from start to completion of treatment - fair outcomes did met criteria for minimally relevant clinical change (i.e. although not as successful as a good or excellent outcome they did respond to treatment); the last table presents efficiency of treatment.

Table 7-4: Consecutive case study of DRS practitioners (7) The effectiveness and efficiency of treatment evaluated by case-type (payment method), activity-level and duration of the musculoskeletal disorder at the initial visit (i.e. confirmatory interests of the study).

	Excellent Outcome	Good Outcome	Fair Outcome	Poor Outcome	Mean Visits	SD ±	Mean Weeks	SD ±
Case-type:								
Medicare (44)	15 (34.1%)	20 (45.5%)	8 (18.2%)	1 (2.3%)	8.7	4.6	4.7	3.0
Private (82)	37 (45.1%)	26 (31.7%)	17 (20.7%)	2 (2.4%)	5.8	3.1	4.0	2.7
Workers Comp (31)	11 (35.5%)	6 (19.4%)	10 (32.3%)	4 (12.9%)	8.3	4.9	4.6	2.8
Motor Vehicle Accident (9)	2 (22.2%)	2 (22.2%)	4 (44.4%)	1 (11.1%)	11.6	6.5	5.3	3.0
Total (166):	65	54	39	8	-	-	-	-
Activity-level: Active (56)	25 (44.6%)	21 (37.5%)	8 (14.3%)	2 (3.6%)	5.9	3.1	4.1	2.8
Idle (31)	11 (35.5%)	5 (16.1%)	12 (38.7%)	3 (9.7%)	7.6	4.5	4.6	2.4
Restricted (21)	5 (23.8%)	6 (28.6%)	8 (38.1%)	2 (9.5%)	9.3	5.7	4.8	3.4
Unknown (58)	24 (41.4%)	22 (37.9%)	11 (19.0%)	1 (1.7%)	7.9	4.7	4.4	2.7
Total (108):	65	54	39	8	-	-	-	-
Duration:								
Acute (< 7 days) 17	9 (52.9%)	5 (29.4%)	3 (17.7%)	0	6.6	3.6	3.7	2.6
Subacute (1-7 wks) 69	31 (44.9%)	24 (34.8%)	10 (14.5%)	4 (5.8%)	6.8	4.4	3.8	2.2
Early Chronic (>7 < 26 wks) 42	14 (33.3%)	14 (33.3%)	12 (28.6%)	2 (4.8%)	7.3	3.9	4.5	2.5
Late Chronic (≥ 26 wks) 38	11 (29.0%)	11 (29.0%)	14 (36.8%)	2 (5.3%)	8.6	5.2	5.4	3.8
Total:	65 (39.2%)	54 (32.5%)	39 (23.5%)	8 (4.8%)	-	-	-	-

Table 7-5: The mean change in numeric pain ratings (0 – 10) are presented.

Outcome Category	Initial Pain Rating				Final Pain Rating			
	Mean	SE Mean	St Dev	Median	Mean	SE Mean	St Dev	Median
Excellent	4.969	0.292	2.352	5.000	0.331	0.0713	0.5747	0.000
Good	5.880	0.315	2.313	5.000	1.657	0.179	1.313	2.000
Fair	5.692	0.373	2.330	5.000	3.667	0.326	2.034	3.500
Poor	4.750	0.796	2.252	4.500	6.000	0.964	2.726	6.500

	Change in Pain Rating						
	Mean	SE Mean	StDev	Median	95 % CI	DF	T-test
Excellent	4.638	0.288	2.321	4.000	4.1 – 5.2	64	16.1
Good	4.222	0.326	2.396	4.000	3.6 – 4.9	53	13.0
Fair	2.026	0.298	1.860	2.000	1.4 – 2.6	38	6.8
Poor	- 1.250	0.491	1.389	-1.000	-2.4 – 0.1	7	- 2.5

The last table (table 7-7) identifies the efficiency of the treatment; note that poor outcomes (i.e. non-responders) are screened-out quickly and those patients seen for the longest time period all responded. This is very important because it can be used to justify continued length of service; it would be fair to criticize a treatment approach that goes on for a long time period with many visits if there isn't an acceptable outcome as a result.

Table 7-6: The mean change in self-rated disability 0-100) per outcome category are presented.

Outcome Category	Initial Disability Rating						Final Disability Rating		
	Mean	SE Mean	Category	Mean	SE Mean	Category	Mean	SE Mean
Excellent	40.03	3.07	24.59	38.50	5.80	0.943	7.544	1.650
Good	46.89	3.16	22.99	50.00	15.63	1.67	12.05	15.0
Fair	56.39	4.30	26.50	59.50	41.81	4.23	25.72	37.00
Poor	55.71	9.74	25.77	51.0	58.20	11.0	27.1	54.5

	Change in Disability Rating						
	Mean	SE Mean	SD ±	Median	95 % CI	DF	T-test
Excellent	34.23	2.88	23.05	30.00	28.5 – 40.0	63	11.9
Good	30.59	2.69	19.41	30.00	25.2 – 36.0	51	11.4
Fair	14.81	3.13	19.06	10.00	8.5 – 21.2	37	4.7
Poor	- 1.67	0.919	2.251	-0.500	- 4.0 – 0.6	6	- 1.8

Table 7-7: Efficiency of treatment outcome is measured by the number of visits required to achieve the outcome.

Outcome	Visits					
	1 – 3 visits	4 – 6 visits	7 – 10 visits	≥ 11 visits	Mean visits	SE
Excellent	16	22	18	9	6.6	4.0
Good	6	24	14	10	7.3	5.0
Fair	4	12	9	14	9.0	5.0
Poor	1	5	2	0	4.9	1.6
Totals:	**27**	**63**	**43**	**33**		
Outcome	Weeks					
	1 – 2 weeks	3 – 6 wks	7 – 12 wks	≥ 13 wks	Mean Weeks	SE
Excellent	17	36	11	1	4.1	2.8
Good	12	34	7	1	4.5	3.0
Fair	7	21	10	1	5.0	2.7
Poor	4	4	0	0	3.1	1.5
Totals:	**40**	**95**	**28**	**3**		

References Chapter 7

Abenhaim L, Rossignol M, Valat JP, et al. The role of activity in the therapeutic management of back pain: report of the international Paris task force on back pain.

Spine 25 (4S): 1S – 33S, 2000.

Bandura, A. Self-efficacy: The exercise of control. WH Freeman and Co., New York, 1997.

Bialosky JE, Bishop MD, Cleland JA. Individual expectation: an overlooked, but pertinent, factor in the treatment of individuals experiencing musculoskeletal pain. Physical Therapy 90 (9): 1345 – 55, 2012.

Edwards RR, Almeida DM, Klick B, Haythornwaite JA, Smith MT. Duration of sleep contributes to next-day pain report in the general population. Pain 137 (1): 202-7, 2008.

Hubble MA, Duncan BL, Miller SD. The Heart & Soul of Change: What Works in Therapy. American Psychological Association, Washington D.C., 1999.

Karas R, McIntosh G, Hall H, et al. The relationship between nonorganic signs and centralization of symptoms in the prediction of return to work for patients with low back pain. Phys Ther 77:354–60, 1997.

Kopp JR, Alexander AH, Turocy RH, et al: The Use of Lumbar Extension in the Evaluation and Treatment of Patients with Acute Herniated Nucleus Pulposus. Clin Orthop 202: 211-218, 1986.

Marin R, Cyhan T, Miklos W: Sleep disturbance in patients with chronic low back pain. Am J Phys Med Rehabil 85:430-435, 2006.

Neck Pain Task Force: The Bone and Joint Decade (2000-2010) Task Force on Neck Pain and Its Associated Disorders. Spine 33 (4S): S1 – S220, 2008

Rath W. Cervical traction: a clinical perspective. Orthopaedic Review, 13(8), 29-48, 1984.

8 MANUAL THERAPY GUIDELINES

Manual therapy is delivered in many different forms, with varying rationales and theoretical models (Vincenzino 2007). These techniques have a mechanical, physiological and/or psychological effect; however, in spite of the many proposed differences in technique and theory, there are many common elements amongst all of the prominent 'schools of thought'. Three common elements are: 1) a system of assessment to identify and characterize the 'lesion' that requires manipulation, 2) the application of force to move the spinal or extremity articulation(s) and/or have a specific biomechanical effect upon the soft tissues, and 3) there is the expectation of an immediate change in signs and/or symptoms as a result of the application of the technique.

This is a basic clinical process that has been in practice since recorded medical history, and (interestingly) many of the manual tools we use today have not changed for hundreds of years (Schiötz and Cyriax 1975). This is currently true for the different 'schools of thought'. When the title and description is removed, the patient's position, the operator's manual contact and line of drive look remarkably similar for supposedly different techniques. It is fascinating how the same, basic biomechanical procedures can have so many different descriptions and explanations (Rath 2002). In this chapter I address guidelines for the indication and application of four general groups of manual therapy techniques: 1) joint mobilization or manipulation, 2) combined performance mobilization, 3) transverse friction massage, and 4) soft-tissue mobilization (stretching).

"First Do No Harm" (Attributed to Hippocrates): The guiding axiom of the Hippocratic Oath, "primum non nocere" or first do no harm, applies to all of healthcare. Most manual therapy techniques are not forceful enough to do any harm, but some are – particularly high velocity techniques to the upper cervical spine (Australian PT Association 1988; Hurwitz 1996; Ernst 2010). However, harm can also be caused by delaying or interfering with natural history (Indahl 1995), enhancing fear avoidance behaviors (Houben 2005a,b), and/or by passive treatment that creates dependencies (Nordin 2001); these factors can negatively influence the patient's expectations, generate unnecessary costs and facilitate disability – generally referred to as iatrogenesis (Pransky 2011). Meader (1994) published in the New England Journal of Medicine that the only remaining people who are healthy are those that have not been worked-up. The selection of patients for manual therapy, the biomechanical forces applied, and the role of these 'time-tested' techniques within the treatment plan requires guidelines to be safe and effective.

Some Definitions of Terms for Manual Therapy

1. Grades of mobilization – there are various grading systems utilized in manual therapy 'schools of thought'. We utilize a simple 3-grade system to identify the biomechanical effect on the joint and/or soft-tissue structure or tissues.

Grade 1 (Mid-range: MR) – the biomechanical force is applied without removing the slack in the joint capsule/ligaments and/or the soft-tissues target for the procedure.

Grade 2 (End Range: ER) – the biomechanical force is applied to the point of removing the slack in the joint capsule/ligaments and/or the soft-tissues target for the procedure but not beyond; i.e. end range elasticity is not challenged.

Grade 3 (End Range Overpressure: EROP) – the biomechanical force is applied to the point of removing the slack in the joint capsule/ligaments and/or the soft-tissue target for the procedure and then additional (controlled) force applied; i.e. end range elasticity is challenged. Ultimately it is the response of the joint to repeated EROP that determines its health (see our functional definition of normal joint motion below).

Figure 8-1: Application of the stress/strain curve for collagen tissue to the grade of mobilization. Grade 1 is the toe region to the left where there is still slack in the tissue. Grade 2 is the very beginning of the elastic region in the middle left region of the curve. Grade 3 is the elastic region and the beginning of the plastic zone to the right side of the   curve.

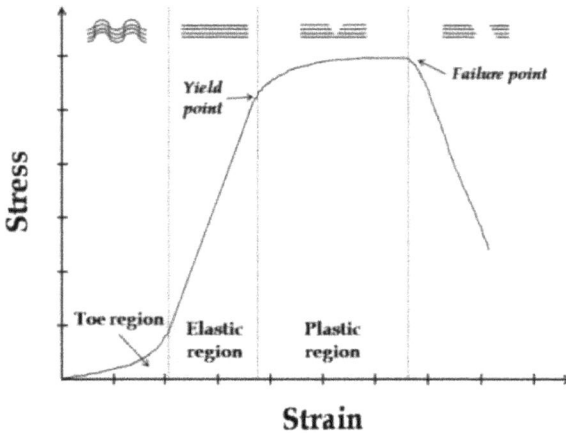

Normal joint motion – the state or condition where the joint can be moved from mid-range to and from end range without pain, have a normal symptom response to progressive (appropriate) overpressure at end range that includes no adverse effect on movement in the opposite and other directions. This status holds up to repeated assessment and is found in all directions that the joint under investigation is designed to move.

2. Types of Mobilization Procedures – mobilizations are any procedure intended to restore and/or improve the quality or quantity of motion. These procedures can be applied to the joints and/or the soft tissues. They can be applied by the therapist (passive technique), the patient (self-mobilization) or some combination. These techniques can be applied slowly or rapidly, intermittently or sustained, gently or aggressively. The following are commonly used terms to describe or identify these procedures:

Joint mobilization – a biomechanical procedure designed to isolate control of the technique to restoring the quality and/or quantity of joint (articular) motion or function.

Soft-tissue mobilization – a biomechanical procedure designed to isolate control of the technique to restoring the quality and/or quantity of soft-tissue extensibility or function.

Combined performance techniques (CPT) – a biomechanical procedure designed to restore the quality and/or quantity of motion due to joint and/or soft-tissue dysfunction that is performed by both the patient and therapist simultaneously.

Transverse friction massage (TFM) – a manual massage procedure applied to the soft-tissues across its longitudinal orientation with the intent of helping to improve the quality and/or quantity of soft-tissue extensibility or function.

Positive transverse friction response – this is the progressive reduction of the patient's relevant symptoms during the application of the massage, followed by an immediate improvement in their relevant sign(s). This response is required to identify the indication for use of these procedures.

Duffy-Rath Definition of Manipulation: "the purposeful and controlled application of biomechanical force(s) to the moving parts of the musculoskeletal system with the intent of relieving relevant signs and symptoms, and restoring physical function".

Manipulative Thrust – this is a small amplitude high velocity pressure at end range. At least one set of mobilization should be performed before the application of a manipulative thrust. These high velocity procedures should be used for Stage II disorders only.

Uncle Ernie's Rule: using the DRS principles of clinical assessment, varying the technique ('fiddle about') before abandoning the use of manual therapy procedures. Especially if the current history suggests that the problem is biomechanical in behavior, the condition is not worsening, and there are positions, movements or activities that make the condition better.

3. Terms to Assess Patient Response to Manual Therapy Procedures –

your system for assessing the response of the patient to the application of manual therapy is critical for safety and effectiveness (Rath 1993); all mobilizations are assessment procedures first and become a treatment procedure only when the correct response is obtained. You assess the symptom response first, the sign response second and the effect on function third.

Stages of assessment - there are three distinct points of assessment when determining the patient's response: 1) RSSx present before application of the procedure, 2) symptom response during the application of the procedure, and 3) RSSx and function response after (as a result of) the application of the procedure. See tables 8-1,2,3 below.

Table 8-1: The possible symptom responses that occur during the application of a manual therapy procedure are determined by the presence or absence of symptoms prior to initiation of the technique.	
Status Prior	**Symptom Response**
No symptoms prior	Either symptoms are produced or there is no effect upon the symptoms
Symptoms prior	Symptoms can increase, decrease, abolish or not be effected.

Increases - this refers to the enhancement of symptoms during a mechanical testing or treatment procedure that were present prior to the performance of the mechanical test or procedure (example: on a visual analog scale it will be X number prior to the test or procedure and X plus during the test or application of the procedure.)

Decreases - this refers to the reduction of symptoms during a mechanical testing or treatment procedure that were present prior to the performance of the mechanical test or procedure (example: on a visual analog scale it will be X number prior to the test or procedure and X minus during the test or application of the procedure.)

Produces - this refers to the development of symptoms during a mechanical testing or treatment procedure that were not present prior to the performance of the mechanical test or procedure (example: on a visual analog scale it will be 0 prior to commencing the mechanical test or procedure, and X during the test or application of the procedure.)

Abolishes - this refers to the removal of symptoms during a mechanical testing or treatment procedure that were present prior to the performance of the mechanical test or procedure (example: on a visual analog scale it will be X prior to commencing the mechanical test or procedure, and 0 during the test or application of the procedure.)

No Effect - this refers to the failure to produce symptoms if not present or to alter symptoms if present during the application of mechanical testing or treatment procedure (example: on a visual analog scale if X prior to the mechanical test or procedure, it remains X during the test or procedure. If 0 prior to the mechanical test or procedure, it remains 0 during the test or procedure.)

Table 8-2: Symptoms that are produced or increased with a manual therapy procedure can be affected at mid-range or at end range; this distinction is important for making a structural prediction and assessing the patient's response. The assessment of symptom response to EROP can be an important tool to distinguish pain during movement vs. end range.	
Symptoms produced or increase during movement (DM)	Symptom effect occurs on the way towards or away from end range and/or there is no progressive increase of 'the' symptoms with increasing overpressure at end range.
Symptoms produced or increase at end range (ER)	Symptom effect occurs at end range and there is a progressive increase of 'the' symptoms with increasing overpressure at end range.

Pain During Movement - this refers to the production or increase of pain in the mid- range of movement; that is, while moving toward or away from the end range with overpressure. This production or increase of pain does NOT continually increase with the progression of force to end range or when progressively increasing amounts of overpressure are applied.

Pain At End Range - refers to the increase or production of pain at the limit of motion which is progressively increased when further amounts of overpressure is applied. This end range pain is increased when progressively increasing amounts of overpressure are applied at end range

Table 8-3: When a biomechanical procedure or activity is repeated or sustained the description of the patient's initial response is determined by the presence or absence of symptoms prior; i.e. using standardized assessment terminology. However, the initial symptom response does not necessarily predict the final response – the result is determined by assessing for change in the response during the procedure or activity, and most importantly any change in the symptoms and signs afterwards – ultimately by any impact on function.

Initial Symptom Response	Possible Responses During the Assessment, Treatment or Activity	Possible Final Responses (As a Result)
Produced	Decreases, Abolishes, Increases, No change	Better – Worse – No Worse
Increased	Decreases, Abolishes, Increases, No change	Better – Worse – No Worse
Abolished	Increases, No change	Better – Worse – No Better
No Effect	Produces, Increases, Decreases, Abolishes, No Change	Better – Worse – In Status Quo

Better - refers to the lasting decrease or abolition of symptoms after the mechanical test or procedure has been applied (example: on a visual analog scale if X was present prior to the application of the mechanical test or treatment procedure, X minus or 0 is the measurement after the test or treatment procedure has ceased.)

No Better - refers to the failure to have a lasting decrease or abolishment of symptoms after the mechanical test or procedure has been applied. Pain that was decreased or abolished during the application of mechanical force returns to the level reported prior to the application of force (example: on a visual analog scale if X was present prior to the application of the mechanical test or treatment procedure, X is the measurement after the test or treatment procedure has ceased.)

Worse - refers to the lasting increase or production of symptoms after the mechanical test or procedure has been applied (example: on a visual analog scale if X was present prior to the application of the mechanical test or treatment procedure, X plus is the measurement after the test or treatment procedure has ceased.)

No Worse - refers to the lack of a lasting increase or production of symptoms after the mechanical test or procedure has been applied. Pain that was increased or produced during the application of mechanical force returns to the level reported prior to the application of force (example: on a visual analog scale if X was present prior to the application of the mechanical test or treatment procedure, X is the measurement after the test or treatment procedure has ceased.)

In Status Quo – the symptoms were not affected during or after the application of the procedure(s).

Paradoxical Pain Responses – term used to describe the situation when the initial response of the patient's symptoms and signs to assessment or treatment procedures is the opposite of the final response. For example: when pain that is increased or produced with movement, positioning or manual therapy procedure at first, with repetition causes the condition to improve.

Centralization of pain – coined by McKenzie (1981), defined as: "centralisation is the phenomenon whereby as a result of the performance of certain repeated movements or the adoption of certain positions, radiating symptoms originating from the spine and referred distally, are caused to move proximally towards the mid line of the spine". Donelson et. al. (1990) in his first study of this phenomenon provided the following definition: "centralization refers to a rapid change in the perceived location of pain from a distal or peripheral location to a more proximal or central one". In a later prospective study of centralization the definition was refined to include the abolition of mid-line pain alone and/or the proximal migration of pain in response to repeated end range movements (Donelson 1997).

In the DRS we distinguished centralization of pain from the centralization phenomenon. The former describes the change in symptom location only. The later requires not only the symptom change, but also improvement in joint motion and a lasting improvement in a weight bearing/functional environment. We made this distinction because the centralization phenomenon was associated with a better and more rapid outcome in our ongoing outcome assessments.

Peripheralization of pain – the opposite of centralization in response to repeated or sustained mechanical loading; indicating a worsening of the clinical condition and need to stop or avoid those activities or treatment procedures for at least the time being.

Directional preference - Donelson (1991) was the first to use the term directional preference in a study investigating the effect of end range flexion and extension movements on pain intensity and location in patients with low back and referred pain. It was stated that "nearly one half of the subjects had a clear directional preference based on the presence of centralization. Forty percent improved with extension and worsened with flexion, whereas 7 % improved with flexion and worsened with extension." This was an important step towards making more clinicians and researchers aware that the tactics of an exercise and/or manual therapy program can be critical to an optimal and rapid response. Since this publication the term "directional preference" has been commonly used to describe groups of patients with ARMSD that can rapidly improve with treatment provided it is properly directed, while the opposite (aggravating) direction is avoided or controlled.

Duffy-Rath Traffic Light Tool – this was developed to train both patients and clinicians to assess the responses of the patient's RSSx to repeated examination procedures, exercise, manual therapy and other treatment tools. A Red light indicates when the procedures should be stopped immediately, a green light indicates a clear and unambiguous improvement and the indication to continue, and the yellow light indicates the possibility of positive or negative change (or no change), hence the need to be cautious until a clear pattern of response emerges (see table 8-4 below).

Guidelines for Application of Joint Mobilization/Manipulation Procedures

Joint mobilization and manipulation procedures are applied when there is a relevant loss of joint motion with the intent of restoring both quality and/or quantity of motion. These tools need to be used with specificity, good reasoning and as a means of helping the patient to achieve self-efficacy.

Table 8-4: Duffy-Rath Musculoskeletal Traffic-light Tool© In 1985 Wayne and Jean developed the 'Musculoskeletal Traffic-light Tool' as a guideline to help the clinician and the patient assess response to assessment, manual therapy and therapeutic procedures.	
RED LIGHT (STOP)	Symptom pattern is expanding. Symptoms are progressively increasing in response to a consistent or diminishing amount of loading. The increase or production of symptoms persists after the load is removed. There is the production or increase of relevant clinical signs (movement loss, neural tension, neurologic, function intolerance etc.)
YELLOW LIGHT (PROCEED CAUTIOUSLY)	Symptoms are being produced or increased, but are not progressive, are not persisting after the load is removed and are not associated with a production or increase of relevant signs. Signs and symptoms are reduced or eliminated with the application of load, but this improvement does not last upon reassessment.
GREEN LIGHT (GO)	Symptoms are contracting, decreasing or are eliminated. Relevant clinical signs are lessening or eliminated. The improvement in symptoms and signs lasts after the load is removed, including with functional reassessment.

Classic joint mobilization techniques performed by the therapist require one of the articular surfaces to be stabilized (usually proximal) and the other manually moved. The arthrokinematics is defined in relation to the concave articular surface; this is called the **"treatment plane"** – a parallel line across the distal end of the concave articular surface. Therefore a glide is movement parallel to the treatment plane and a traction is 90 degrees perpendicular to the treatment plan and separates the articular surfaces (compression approximates the surfaces), etc. This language is used to describe the line of drive of the forces used to manually restore motion at the articular level.

The following are guidelines for application of therapist mobilization/manipulation procedures:

- Be conservative with the application of biomechanical forces. Always start gently and don't progress any further than the patient's response allows, or any further than what is required to achieve the desired clinical effect (i.e. the 'least force rule').
- A joint mobilization procedure begins in mid-range and when the response is appropriate proceeds to end range and eventually to enough overpressure (no more than necessary) to determine the end range response with the intent of restoring normal movement.

- Include the patient in the decision-making process, and receive consent before proceeding. Provide an explanation for the procedure regarding: method, intent, expectations and options.
- Identify the desired effect on the RSSx, and relate the use of the procedure to function and self-efficacy.
- Analyze symptom response first, sign response second, and ultimately determine the effect on function as a result. Use the traffic-light analogy.
- When symptoms are constant, the first goal is to convert to intermittent. Stay in mid-range until it is certain that proceeding further is not contraindicated.
- When symptoms are unstable intermittent, the first goal to convert to stable intermittent. Start with the same approach as with constant symptoms, but there is greater probability that you can progress safely to end range when there is an unequivocal directional preference.
- When symptoms are stable intermittent, the goal is to abolish them or eliminate their interference with activity and function. You need to proceed to end range in order to determine the true mechanical nature of the problem.
- When symptoms are present prior to the application of the joint mobilization procedure the segmental level(s) that reduces or abolishes the symptoms is the target level(s).
- When symptoms are not present prior to the application of the joint mobilization procedure the segmental level(s) that reduces or abolishes the symptoms with the movement (i.e. the relevant sign) is the target level(s). At first this is often the level(s) that initially produces 'the' symptoms, but then progressively improves with repetition (i.e. paradoxical pain response). Follow guidelines for assessment of response.

Analyzing the Performance of the Manual Techniques

The performance of a manual therapy procedure can be assessed according to the following 7 criteria; this provides a means to problem-solve difficulties in learning a technique as well as serving as the basis for developing a method to rate a clinician's clinical performance:

1. **Patient position** – is the patient position comfortable and appropriate for the specific application of force with good therapist biomechanics?
2. **Therapist position** – is the therapist position appropriate for the specific application of force and the use of good biomechanics?
3. **Contact** – is the contact comfortable and effective to achieve the intended effect of the procedure?
4. **Line of drive** (direction/application of force) – are the applied forces going in the correct direction to achieve the intended biomechanical effect?
5. **Control of technique** – does the therapist demonstrate the ability to appropriately and effectively control the force used to achieve the intended effect of the procedure?
6. **Comfort** – is the application of the technique comfortable and appropriate, encouraging patient confidence and relaxation?
7. **Assessment of response** - does the therapist effectively assess the patient's response to the application of the technique?

Joint Cavitation & the Biomechanical Forces of Spinal Manipulation

A manual therapist needs to have a thorough knowledge of their biomechanical tools, especially high velocity techniques applied to the spine. As previously mentioned in this chapter, the cervical spine is at greatest risk for adverse response to manipulative thrust (Hurwitz 1996; DiFabio 1999; Tseng 2002; Ernst 2010). We need to know the mechanism and relevance of the audible pop (i.e. cavitation), and the magnitude, amplitude and kinematics of the various techniques. We advocate for the use of the progression of force concept proposed by McKenzie (1989) – a close and objective look at the magnitude of forces applied with thrust techniques and the mechanism of joint cavitation makes the need for a careful assessment (selection) system apparent.

The progression of force concept proposes that the manual therapist should view the application of mobilization/manipulation to the spinal joints as a spectrum of force that starts with patient self-mobilization in mid-range and culminates with high velocity thrust at end range. It is suggested that this renders the application of thrust techniques safer (i.e. you don't progress the force when lesser amounts create an adverse effect) and reserves these technique for those patients who need them (i.e. when the signs and symptoms are eliminated with lesser force why provide more). The emphasis is placed on the assessment of the patient's response (symptoms and signs) all along the course of this spectrum – an approach that we have illustrated throughout this book to have the greatest evidence-based support. This enables the clinician to more reliably identify the level of the mechanical lesion and indication for more force; this also encourages the treatment strategy to focus on patient education for self-efficacy.

Manipulative therapists and the public put too much emphasis on the audible pop; this focus is distracting to the larger, more important issues facing clinical management of MSD; i.e. optimizing patient selection, the long-term effect of treatment on activity and the elimination of the need for further, progressive healthcare intervention. The noise associated with spinal manipulation is the result of the sudden formation and collapse of low-pressure, nitrogen bubbles in the synovial fluids of the joint; i.e. cavitation (Roston 1949; Unsworth 1971). These noises can be rendered in any joint regardless of the presence or absence of a joint dysfunction or disorder. Ross et. al. (2004) demonstrated that a skilled manipulator has a 50/50 chance of isolating the cavitation effect to a specific spinal level. Making the audible release the 'holy grail' of manipulation (Rosner 2004) is out of focus with all evidence regarding diagnosis and treatment of ARSD. I agree with the physical therapy-based position proposed by Flynn et. al. (2003) that the "audible pop is not necessary for successful spinal high-velocity thrust manipulation".

Measuring the Force of High Velocity Thrust – the amount of force transmitted to the spinal joint is a product of the magnitude and velocity of the technique. Velocity is the critical factor for two reasons; 1) increasing speed of the force applied amplifies the force significantly, and 2) high velocity creates a momentary 'out-of-control' element to the technique. The combination of these two factors increases the risk for injury when the wrong joint is manipulated in the wrong direction – a major reason for the progression of force concept.

By definition, a thrust technique is a small amplitude procedure with a high velocity. The emphasis should be small (controlled) amplitude; a psychomotor skill an experienced manual therapist has mastered.

Referring back to the stress – strain curve, these techniques take place in the elastic/early plastic zone - this is why they can be (potentially) dangerous, even in the hands of an experienced and manually skilled practitioner. Increasing velocities of manipulative thrust have been measured to increase displacement fivefold (Colloca 2006).

These techniques take the target joint to end range (i.e. remove the slack in the joint) and first explore intermittent overpressure. Once a green light is obtained a high velocity force is applied; provided the therapist does not release the slack that was removed and he/she has full control of the depth of the force the amplitude of the technique remains small and controlled. However, many inexperienced and unskilled therapist release the slack that was removed in their effort to generate the velocity of the thrust – this generates larger amplitude, higher velocity forces. This results in loss of control of the force and greater likelihood of injury by bringing the tissues to the failure point. This is a reason for clinically supervised training when learning thrust techniques, practicing on inanimate objects to gain the psychomotor skill, and then using the progression of force concept in determining level, direction and need with patients.

The large forces generated by these techniques are the result of the high velocity. The largest forces are applied to the lumbar spine and the least to the neck, but the magnitudes are significant in all regions. Kawchuk et. al. (1992) measured an average of 117.7 N (±15.6N) peak force for cervical manipulative technique. Thoracic manipulation registered an average peak force of 238.2 N with a P-A thrust to transverse processes T3-10 (Herzog 2001). Triano et. al. (1997) investigated three different lumbar techniques; 1) mamillary push (MP), 2) hypothenar ischial (HI) and long lever lumbar (LLL). The average peak force was 495.5N (MP), 515.5N (HI) and 384.7N (LLL). He reports that the loads were found to be more complex than anticipated, influenced by patient posture and position.

Conway et. al. (1993) presented the results of an interesting study that measured the force required to cause cavitation with an extension manipulation of T-4 by one clinician with 10 subjects. The average preload force (i.e. taking up the slack) was 145N (±54N), average peak force 400N (±118N) and cavitation occurred at an average force of 364N (±106N). The difference between preload and peak force is significant and this is where injury with high velocity technique can occur. The application of this amount of force should never be casually administered, but when applied needs to be at the correct level, in the correct direction and for the correct reason. It is curious to find that cavitation always occurred with less than the peak force (table 8-5).

Table 8-5: T-4 P-A thrust by one clinician, 10 subjects, enough force to produce cavitation (Conway 1993).		
Parameter	Mean	SD
Preload force	145 N	54 N
Peak Force	400 N	118 N
Force of cavitation	364 N	106 N
Time to peak force	150 ms	77 ms
Time to cavitation	116 ms	39 ms
N = unit of force that would give a mass of 1 Kg an acceleration of one meter per second per second		

The bottom-line is that these forces are significant and need to be used judiciously. I advocate that a skilled thruster of joints must first be a skilled mobilizer of joints. Since the introduction of 'mobilization with movement' by Mulligan the need to employ high velocity thrust has diminished. We encourage you to develop these psychomotor skills, but operate guided by the progression of force concept (i.e. least force required rule).

Combined Performance Technique Procedures

These procedures involve the active participation of both the patient and therapist. The therapist applies a sustained mobilization or soft-tissue technique and the patient actively performs the movement or function you are attempting to restore.

McKenzie (1981) was the first therapist I encountered using these combined performance procedures, but he only did this with manual overpressure during the 'Press-up' (prone extension movement) – it quickly became an important part of my lumbar assessment and treatment routine. We then started experimenting with combined traction with extension of the cervical and lumbar spine with good results. However, it was our experiences with Mulligan that started in 1984 that stimulated us to incorporate this into our system as a foundational procedure. Mulligan's publication of 'Mobilization with Movement' (1999) popularized the use of these techniques to the entire musculoskeletal system – a major advancement in manual therapy. Jean and I helped introduce Mulligan to the United States in 1985 and strongly encourage manual therapist to become familiar with his treatment techniques; they are crucial to both assessment and treatment.

You need to follow the same assessment guidelines for the application of joint (or soft-tissue) mobilization. However, because of the combination of therapist technique and patient movement, there are two basic components to these procedures to assess and control:

Therapist technique – this is the mobilization performed by the therapist to the joint or soft-tissue under treatment. This is a glide, traction and/or rotation to the joint; or a pressure, TFM or stretch to the soft-tissue. The grade of force should be consistent throughout the entire patient movement or task (beginning to end); adjusted according to the patient's response – follow guidelines.

Patient technique – this is the movement or task performed by the patient; i.e. the sign you are attempting to eliminate, or the function you are attempting to restore. When the response is appropriate, the patient movement or task should be repeated and progressed – follow guidelines. When a successful technique is found, convert to a self-mobilization procedure and connect to instructions for biomechanical control.

Transverse Friction Massage Procedures

Our use of transverse friction massage (TFM) is a modification of the techniques first identified by Cyriax (1982; 1984). The first, most essential step is to carefully identify that the pain generator lies within the soft-tissues; i.e. muscle, tendon, bursa, ligament etc. The second step is to determine if the site of the lesion is within manual reach through careful palpation. A TFM is attempted if you find a spot(s) that reproduces 'the' symptoms and/or is exquisitely tender (compare to the other side when possible and/or needed). At this point you apply the TFM looking for a '**Positive Transverse Friction Response**', to determine if this treatment procedure is indicated. The following describes the process and response:

Identify the structure to massage, and place enough pressure to elicit 'the' pain (don't press harder, especially at first). Apply a cross friction movement, maintaining the exact same pressure, across the fibers of the structure you are massaging. The symptoms should not increase, if they do ease-up on the pressure (if that does not help, stop). The first indication of a positive response is that the symptoms begin to lessen during the application of the massage. Continue until the symptom response stops, or stops lessening. The second assessment is to reassess the most relevant sign(s) – if there is significant improvement and/or the sign(s) is temporarily abolished you have achieved a positive transverse friction response. This is an indication that this tool is highly likely to be useful to help gain control over the patient's RSSx.

When a positive response has been achieved you should teach the patient and/or 'significant other' to perform the TFM at home; include clear guidelines, start conservatively and instruct them to use heat prior/ice afterwards PRN. This treatment tool is almost exclusively used with our remodeling treatment strategy, so it is applied during the process of regaining soft-tissue extensibility and joint ROM and/or normalizing muscle contraction response – TFM is an important adjunct tool to help the process of restoring function and activity tolerance. The patient experiences a consistent (positive) cause and effect with the TFM and this can be very encouraging and important to building musculoskeletal self-efficacy.

A **progressive TFM** is applied when the patient has demonstrated a consistent improvement over the course of at least 1 – 2 weeks of treatment with the massage technique, but progress has stalled (i.e. the relevant sign has not cleared). In addition there has to be no evidence of any adverse reaction to the technique; e.g. persistent soreness from the manual pressure, contusion, etc. – in other words, they tolerate the technique well. At this point the massage can be progressed in one of two ways: 1) by gradually increasing the depth of the massage as the symptom response to the technique abolishes, or 2) placing the target tissue or structure under tension (e.g. on stretch, or a sustained contraction of the muscle etc.) while performing the technique. This later progression falls within the concept of combined performance technique in our system.

Soft-tissue Mobilization (Stretching)

Range of motion or 'stretching' procedures have been an important treatment and prevention tool since the inception of Physical Therapy. Loss of soft-tissue extensibility is a common finding with MSD; these signs can have direct or indirect relevance and/or can be a predisposing factor to a cumulative disorder. Consequently stretching procedures represent a bulk of the soft-tissue mobilization procedures employed in our system.

We follow the same guidelines of assessment as described for joint mobilization techniques: assess the symptom response first, sign response second and then impact on function last. Use the DR traffic light tool as a guide – start conservatively and progress as needed once the patient demonstrates tolerance to the procedures.

All stretching techniques need to be performed properly with an emphasis on biomechanical control. When the intent is to restore or preserve joint ROM remove any interference from external, multi-joint soft-tissues. When the intent is to restore or preserve elasticity of soft-tissues be certain to isolate the effects of the procedure and prevent compensatory joint motion. When the intent is to reduce or eliminate adverse neural or root tension be extremely conservative in the initiation of these procedures until tolerance is clear and unambiguous.

Intermittent or Sustained Stretching

The question of whether or not to sustain a stretch remains an issue of controversy and confusion. The following discussion presumes that we are addressing the need to restore extensibility to a shortened/contracted soft-tissue or joint capsule/ligament; i.e. there is no evidence of internal derangement or a tracking problem in the joint, this is not early post trauma or surgery, or an active inflammatory disease process etc.

To start, collagen tissue can be elongated only by removing slack and applying an end range load. Flowers and LaStrayo (1994) demonstrated that the 'total end range time' has predictive value to improving passive range of motion – this is consistent with collagen and scar tissue research. However, the patient needs to tolerate the stretching procedure in order to respond to the treatment and want to continue with the remodeling process.

Consistent with the progression of force concept, an intermittent stretch imparts less force (stress/strain) than a sustained stretch provided the magnitude of the force is the same. This is because the time at end range is obviously less; consequently the quantity of force is less and consequently so is the viscoelastic effect of the procedure. This might ultimately (but not definitely) be a limiting factor to the potential benefit of an intermittent stretching technique – however the patient's response comes first, and much of the research is applicable to muscle and scar tissue stretching - and with many cumulative disorders this is not applicable. It is best to start conservatively, prove tolerance and then gradually progress your techniques toward a specific goal achievement.

Manual Therapy Guidelines Summary

Manual therapy is an extremely important component of musculoskeletal assessment and treatment; the knowledge, skills and experience obtained can then be applied to the development of prevention tools. There needs to be a system to determine who requires the application of specific techniques, and a system to evaluate the patient's response that renders the treatment both safe and effective. We emphasized the importance of the 'progression of force' concept and the assessment of the patient's symptoms first, signs second, and impact on function third. We encourage the clinician to begin conservatively, prove patient tolerance and benefit to the application of the procedure and then progress as needed.

Manual therapy is a fun and exciting component of musculoskeletal care and we look forward to helping you develop and augment your manual skills. However, it is a tool that has short-term impact and is most effective when combined with exercise and education (Bronfort 2001; Evans 2002; Assendelft 2003). This is consistent with the general philosophy of the Duffy-Rath System©, but it is also commonsense when considering the long-term concerns for patients with MSD.

References Chapter 8

Assendelft WJ, Morton SC, Yu EI, et. al. Spinal manipulative therapy for low back pain. A meta-analysis of effectiveness relative to other therapies. The Cochrane Back Review Group, Toronto, Ontario, Canada. Ann Inter Med: 138 (11): 871-81, 2003.

Australian Physiotherapy Association. Protocol for pre-manipulative testing of the cervical spine, 1988.

Bronfort G, Evans R, Nelson B, et. al. A randomized clinical trial of exercise and spinal manipulation for patients with chronic neck pain. Spine 26 (7): 788 -99, 2001

Colloca CJ, Keller TS, Harrison DE, et. al. Spinal manipulation force and duration affect vertebral movement and neuromuscular responses. Clinical Biomechanics 21 (3): 254-262, 2006.

Conway P, Herzog W, Zhang Y, Hasler E, Ladly K. Forces required to cause cavitation during spinal manipulation of the thoracic spine. Clin Biomech 8 (4):210-4, 1993.

Cyriax J: Textbook of Orthopaedic Medicine: Vol I. Diagnosis of Soft Tissue Lesions, 8th Edition. London, Bailliere Tindall, 1982.

Cyriax, J, Coldham M. Textbook of Orthopedic Medicine Vol II: Treatment by Manipulation and Massage and Injection, 11th Edition. Bailliere Tindall, London 1984.

DiFabio RF. Manipulation of the cervical spine: risks and benefits. Phy Ther 79 (1): 50-65, 1999.

Donelson R, Silva G, Murphy K. Centralization phenomenon. Its usefulness in evaluating and treating referred pain. Spine 15(3):211–3, 1990.

Donelson R, Grant W, Kamps C, et al. Pain response to sagittal end-range spinal motion. A prospective, randomized, multicentered trial. Spine 16(6S):S206–12, 1991.

Donelson R, Aprill C, Medcalf R, et al. A prospective study of centralization of lumbar and referred pain. A predictor of symptomatic discs and annular competence. Spine. 22 (10):1115–22, 1997.

Ernst E. Deaths after chiropractic: a review of published cases. Int J Clin Pract 64 (10): 1162-65, 2010.

Evans R, Bronfort G, Nelson B, Goldsmith CH. Two-year follow-up of a randomized clinical trial of spinal manipulation and two types of exercise for patients with chronic neck pain. Spine 27 (21): 2383-89, 2002.

Flowers KR, LaStayo P. Effect of total end range time on improving passive range of motion. J Hand Ther 7 (3): 150-7, 1994.

Flynn TW, Fritz JM, Wainner RS, Whitman JM. The audible pop is not necessary for successful spinal high-velocity thrust manipulation in individuals with low back pain. Arch Phys Med Rehabil 84:1057-60, 2003.

Furlan AD, Brosseau L, Imamura M, Irvin E. Massage for low-back pain: a systematic review within the framework of the Cochrane Collaboration Review Group. Spine 27 (17): 1896-1910, 2002)

Herzog W, Kats B, Symons B. Effective forces transmitted by high-speed, low-amplitude thoracic manipulation. Spine 26: 2105-2110, 2001.

Houben RM, Gijsen A, Peterson J, de Jong PJ, Vlaeyen JW. Do health care providers' attitudes towards back pain predict their treatment recommendations? Differential predictive validity of implicit and explicit attitude measures Pain 114:491–8, 2005a.

Houben RM, Ostelo RW, Vlaeyen JW, Wolters PM, Peters M, Stomp-van den Berg SG. Health care providers' orientations towards common low back pain predict perceived harmfulness of physical activities and recommendations regarding return to normal activity. Eur J Pain 9:173–83, 2005b.

Hurwitz EL, Aker PD, Adams AH, et. al. Manipulation and mobilization of the cervical spine. A systematic review of the literature. Spine 21 (15): 1746-59, 1996.

Indahl A, Velund L, Reikeraas O: Good prognosis for low back pain when left untampered: a randomized clinical trial. Spine 20 (4): 473-477, 1995.

Kawchuk GN, Herzog W, Hasler EM. Forces generated during spinal manipulative therapy of the cervical spine: a pilot study. J Manipulative Physiol Ther 15 (5): 275-8, 1992.

McKenzie R A The Lumbar Spine. Mechanical diagnosis and therapy Spinal Publications, Waikanae, New Zealand, 1981.

McKenzie RA: A Perspective on Manipulative Therapy. Physiotherapy 75 (8): 440-444, 1989.

Meador CK. The last well person. NEJM 330 (6): 440-41, 1994.

Mulligan BR. Manual Therapy: "Nags", "Snags", MWMs" etc. 3rd Edition Plane View Services, Wellington, New Zealand, 1999.

Nordin M 2000 International society of the study of the lumbar spine presidential address: backs to work: some reflections. Spine 26 (8): 851-856, 2001

Pransky G, Borkan JM, Young AE, Cherkin DC. Are we making progress? The tenth international forum for primary care research on low back pain. Spine 36 (19): 1608-14, 2011.

Rath W. Standardization of terms used in the assessment of pain/symptom responses when mechanical forces are applied to the musculoskeletal system of the human body. McKenzie Institute Newsletter, US. 1 (4), 25 – 30, 1993.

Rath W. Spinal manipulation and the prevention of dysfunction and disability. APTA Combined Sections Meeting, Orthopaedic Section, San Diego Convention Center, Boston, MA, February 23, 2002.

Rosner A. Cavitaion Emptor: tracking the holy grail of manipulation. Dynamic Chiropractic 22 (19): 1-4, 2004.

Ross JK, Bereznick DE, David E, McGill SM. Determining cavitation location during lumbar and thoracic spinal manipulation: is spinal manipulation accurate and specific? Spine 29(13): 1452-57, 2004.

Roston JB, Haines RW. Cracking in the metacarpophalangeal joint. J Anat 81: 165-73, 1949.

Schiotz EH, Cyriax J. Manipulation: Past and Present. London, Heinemann, 1975.

Triano J, Schultz AB Loads transmitted during lumbosacral spinal manipulative therapy. Spine 22: 1955-64, 1997.

Tseng SH, Lin SM, Chen Y, Wang CH. Ruptured cervical disc after spinal manipulation therapy. Spine 27 (3): E80-82, 2002.

Unsworth A, Dowson D, Wright V. Cracking joints: a bioengineering study of cavitation in the metacarpophalangeal joint. Ann Rheum Dis 30 (4): 348-58, 1971.

Vicenzino B, Paungmali A, Teys P Mulligan's mobilizations-with-movement, positional faults and pain relief: current concepts from a critical review of the literature. Manual Therapy 12 (2): 98 – 108, 2007.

9 STATUS POST TRAUMA

Thankfully the majority of MSD are not the result of blunt trauma, however when this is the mechanism of onset special clinical considerations are immediately present. The greatest concern is for serious pathology that contraindicates physical therapy and requires medical/surgical attention. Additionally, most blunt trauma requires diagnostic imaging and/or special diagnostic testing. The musculoskeletal therapist needs to be familiar with evidence-based methods for screening, special regional considerations and 'on-guard' for the patient's best interests. Prior to addressing these regional issues we need to review basic concepts of tissue healing and repair.

Phases of Healing and Tissue Repair

Injury is always followed by repair; a biological phenomenon and imperative that science is unveiling to the benefit of treatment and prevention. Traumatic injuries are the result of high velocity and high magnitude loading that suddenly bring connective tissues to the limit of extensibility and beyond. The resulting musculoskeletal damage involves the soft tissues only or includes the bones – in either case the repair response begins immediately and is defined by 3 general phases: 1) inflammation (exudative phase), 2) proliferation (fibroblastic phase) and 3) remodeling (maturation phase). The timeline for these 3 phases is generally about 3 days for phase 1, up to 3 – 4 weeks for phase 2 and ongoing for phase 3. This maturation phase can take months and years to reach potential depending on the tissue(s) involved, extent of the damage, the presence of confounding factors, the management strategy adopted and the patient's beliefs and behaviors.

The inflammatory phase initiates a series of biochemical reactions that stop the bleeding (platelets), clean-up and protect the wound (neutrophils), and attract the fibroblasts (macrophages) which are essential to repair. The proliferative phase is where fibroblastic activity peaks to initiate angiogenesis, epithelialization and collagen formation.

This phase concludes when the breakdown and synthesis of collagen equalizes. The final phase can go on for days/weeks or months/years depending on the severity of the injury; characterized by a heightened rate of collagen production and breakdown. Collagen reorganizes along lines of tension, so appropriate and progressive activity is critical to quality repair during this phase of healing. Crosslinks are critical to mechanical strength of the collagen, but excessive linkage interferes with normal function.

These phases of repair have characteristics that are unique to the tissues involved and that are relevant to time frames and expected degree of functional recovery. Tendon, ligament, articular cartilage and bone for example have different cellular and biologic processes to consider (Kalfas 2001; Buckwalter 2002; Sharma 2006; Keramaris 2008; Chamberlain 2009; Mihoefer 2009; Hsu 2010). And ultimately, once in the chronic stage of maturation there are the same biologic and behavioral issues that influence the recovery from and/or prevention of cumulative strain and degenerative MSD. In the long run these factors have the greatest influence on recovery from trauma and/or orthopaedic surgery.

Some Regional Considerations

Blunt Trauma to the Neck

Nordin et. al. (2008) provides an excellent overview for this topic related to assessment of neck pain disorders. This is a primary resource and I suggest reviewing the article directly. Motor vehicle accidents, bicycle accidents, sports injuries and falls with head impact are the most common scenarios with these injuries. The first concern is to screen for serious injury; e.g. fracture, dislocation, spinal cord or brain injury. There are 3 evidence-based screening tools you should be familiar with: 1) Glasgow coma scale, 2) Canadian C-spine rule (CCR) and 3) the NEXUS low risk criteria (NLC).

Glasgow Coma Scale (GCS) – this tool is used to rank the severity of head injuries (Teadale 1974; 1976; 1978; Rowley 1991). There are three general categories; eye opening response, verbal response and motor response. Each category has multiple criteria and an assigned number of points. The points assigned for each of the three criteria are totaled with a maximum of 15 points (mild head injury) and a minimum of 3 points (severe head injury = ≤ 8) – see table below:

Table 9-1: the Glasgow Coma Scale (GCS); the lower the score the more serious the head injury.					
Eye Opening Response	Pts	**Verbal Response**	Pts	**Motor Response**	Pts
Spontaneous – open with blinking at baseline	4	Oriented	5	Obeys commands for movement	6
		Confused conversation, but able to answer questions	4		
To verbal stimuli, command, speech	3			Purposeful movement to painful stimuli	5
To pain only (not applied to face)	2	Inappropriate words	3	Withdraws in response to pain	4
		Incomprehensible speech	2		
No response	1	No response	1	Flexion in response to pain (decorticate posturing)	3
				Extension response in response to pain (decerebrate posturing)	2
				No response	1
Severe head injury = GCS ≤ 8 pts. Moderate head injury = GSC 9 – 12 pts. Mild head injury = GCS 13 – 15 pts.					

In general patients with blunt head/neck trauma with a GCS of 15 are considered to be low risk and the need for diagnostic imaging can be assessed using the Canadian C-spine rule (CCR) and/or the NEXUS low-risk criteria (NLC). Validity of these tools has been evaluated and established in comparison to the gold standard 3-view radiograph; i.e. lateral, A-P and open mouth view (Nordin 2008).

Utilizing the GCS, any patient with a score of ≤ 14 is considered high risk and should be screened with diagnostic imaging. In these cases CT scan has been found to have greater diagnostic accuracy than standard radiographs (Hoffman 2000; Holmes 2005; Nordin 2008). When the GCS is 15 the Canadian C-spine Rule (CCR) or the NEXUS (National Emergency X-radiography Utilization Study) Low-risk Criteria (NLC) are evidenced based tools to determine need for diagnostic imaging.

Canadian C-spine Rule (CCR) – this tool is utilized when the GCS is 15 and the patient's condition is stable enough to assess the need for radiography (Steill 2001; 2003; Kerr 2005; Nordin 2008). There are 3 general categories to be evaluated: 1) High risk factors, 2) Safety of evaluating the patient's neck ROM, and 3) the patient's ability to actively rotate their neck. To understand how the CCR is applied we need to provide further guideline and definitions:

1. Any high risk factor mandates radiography – the presence of high risk factors mandates the need for radiography.

These factors include; age ≥ 65 years, dangerous mechanisms of onset (see table below) or paresthesias in the extremities.

Table 9-2: Dangerous mechanisms (CCR)
Fall ≥ 3 feet or 5 stairs, an axial loading to the head (e.g. diving), a motor vehicle collision at high speed (>100km/hr.) or with rollover, ejection or pushed into traffic; a collision involving motorized recreational vehicle; or bicycle struck or collision.

2.   Any low-risk factor which allows for safe assessment of ROM – the absence of low-risk factors mandates the need for radiography.

These low-risk factors are: simple rear-end MVA (this does not include if pushed into oncoming traffic, hit by bus or large truck, rollover or hit by high speed vehicle), sitting position in ER, ambulatory any time, delayed onset of neck pain, and absence of mid-line cervical tenderness.

3.   Able to actively rotate neck – the inability of the patient to actively rotate their neck ≥ 45 degrees in both directions mandates the need for radiography.

To summarize; if there are no high risk factors, but there are low risk factors that allow for safe assessment of neck motion and the patient is able to rotate their neck ≥ 45 degrees in both directions they do not require an immediate radiograph. All others should, with room for discretion of the attending physician.

NEXUS Low Risk Criteria (NLC) – as with the CCR, this tool is utilized when the GCS is 15 (Hoffman 1992; 2000; Panacek 2001; Dickinson 2004; Dearden 2005; Heffernan 2005). There are 5 criteria and if all are found upon clinical assessment than cervical spine radiography is not required. The 5 criteria are as follows:

- No posterior or midline cervical spine tenderness.
- No evidence of intoxication.
- A normal level of alertness.
- No focal neurological deficit.
- No painful distracting injuries.

There are clarifications for each of the NEXUS criteria that help the physician render an interpretation in determining need for radiography (Hoffman 2000). In general, the CCR is found to be more accurate than the NLC (Stiell 2003; Dickinson 2004), but both are validated tools.

Quebec Task Force Report on Whiplash Associated Disorders (WAD) – this is an excellent and comprehensive investigation of whiplash injuries. A recurrent theme throughout the DRS workshop series is the finding that most MSD, even those of traumatic onset have a favorable natural history. However, when trauma is the mechanism of onset the likelihood of having multiple sources of symptoms increases and if this is not sorted-out and each addressed specifically then treatment failure is also more likely. The table below supports these two concepts.

Table 9-3: Even recovery from whiplash is favorable: approximately half have RTW by 4 weeks and 80 % by 6 months have returned to work. Only 2.9 % remain out of work after one year, with secondary injury a significant factor (Spitzer 1995).			
Duration of Absence	All Subjects	Whiplash Only	Whiplash + Other Injury
1 week	621 (22.1 %)	383 (24.7 %)	238 (18.9 %)
4 weeks	709 (25.2 %)	360 (23.2 %)	349 (27.7 %)
8 weeks	422 (15.0 %)	223 (14.4 %)	199 (15.8 %)
26 weeks	542 (19.3 %)	317 (20.5 %)	235 (17.9 %)
52 weeks	435 (15.5 %)	238 (15.3 %)	197 (15.6 %)
> 52 weeks	81 (2.9 %)	30 (1.9 %)	51 (4.1 %)

Blunt Trauma to the Thoracic and Lumbar Spine & Pelvis

Bagley (2006) reports the incidence of blunt trauma affecting the thoracic and lumbar spine to be small (i.e. 2 – 3%), however these injuries can represent up to 40 – 50% of spinal injuries that result in neurologic deficit. As with the cervical spine, computed tomography has been found to have greater diagnostic accuracy than plain radiographs (Campbell 1995; Sheridan 2003; Watura 2004; Herzog 2004; Berry 2005). However, there is a legitimate concern for radiation exposure that the physician must weigh in their decision to choose the most appropriate imaging procedure (Frus 2004). Blunt trauma to the pelvis usually involves a major accident and is a life threatening event when there is haemodynamic instability (Geeraerts 2007). Again, computed tomography is the more reliable and accurate choice for diagnostic imaging and have replaced x-rays in most all cases of blunt trauma to the pelvis (Guillamondegui 2002; Kessel 2007).

Considerations with Shoulder Trauma

Compression fracture of the posterolateral humeral head (Hill-Sachs lesion) with anterior dislocation of the glenohumeral joint is an important complication that can be overlooked, and is likely to progress and contribute to recurrent incidents (Cetik 2007). The Stryker notch view x-ray had been the method of choice for many years, however sonography has proven to be more accurate (Čičak 1998) – detection of a Hill-Sachs lesion has good inter-rater reliability (Sasyniuk 2007). These lesions are often accompanied by a tear to the anterior-inferior labrum, commonly called a Bankart lesion. These are indications for the need to surgically repair. Axillary nerve injury is a consideration with traumatic GHJ dislocation.

Blunt trauma due to lateral impact to the shoulder is associated with mid-shaft clavicle, rib and scapular fractures but can cause a posterior sternoclavicular dislocation which is a life-threatening situation (Laffosee 2010). This is sometimes referred to as scapular-clavicular-thoracic syndrome. Not something likely to be seen in physical therapy undiagnosed, but it is good to be aware of the biomechanics and potential consequences.

With all blunt trauma injuries to the shoulder, there is the possibility for brachial plexus injury – the most common are traction injuries; i.e. where the head and neck are moved away from the involved shoulder. The upper root connections (C5,6) are typically affected when the injury occurs with the arm at the side; when the arm is abducted overhead the lower root connections (C8, T1) are typically affected. The lower plexus lesions are more common; in part this is thought to be due to the absence of a transverse radicular ligament to resist the traction force in the lower roots.

Acromioclavicular joint injuries occur with direct impact to the shoulder. The Rockwood system is used to describe the severity and characteristics of the ACJ injury, distinguishing six grades (see table below). The injury involves the soft tissues, consequently magnetic resonance imaging has been found to be most accurate and informative (Alyas 2008; Nemec 2011).

Table 9-4: The Rockwood grading system for ACJ injuries

Structure	Type 1	Type 2	Type 3	Type 4	Type 5	Type 6 (rare)
AC Ligament	Mild sprain	Ruptured	Ruptured	Ruptured	Ruptured	Ruptured
CC Ligament	intact	Sprain	Ruptured	Ruptured	Ruptured	Ruptured
Joint Capsule	Intact	Ruptured	Ruptured	Ruptured	Ruptured	Ruptured
Deltoid	Intact	Min detach	Detached	Detached	Detached	Detached
Trapezius	Intact	Min detach	Detached	Detached	Detached	Detached
Clavicle	Not elevated	Elevated but not above superior border acromion	Superior to acromion – coracoclavicular distance < 2X normal	Displaced posteriorly into trapezius	Marked elevation – coracoclavicular distance > 2X normal (e.g. > 25mm)	Inferior displaced behind coracobrachialis and biceps tendons

Elbow Trauma

Traumatic fracture and dislocation of the elbow are common; dislocation of the elbow is second only to the shoulder in the general population and the most common in pediatrics (Kuhn 2008). There is evidence that radiologic investigation may not be necessary when the patient has full active ROM, particularly full extension (Lampraikis 2007;

Appelboam 2008) – in many cases a plain radiograph is adequate to establish an accurate diagnosis (Godefroy 2007; Sans 2008). MR imaging provides accurate assessment of the soft-tissues.

Most dislocations occur as the result of a fall on an outstretched arm, but can also occur with high velocity impact. Simple dislocations are soft tissue injuries and can occur in any direction; posterior is most frequent. Complex dislocations include fractures, most commonly involving the radial head and coronoid process – sometimes referred to as the 'terrible triad'. Restoration of full motion and recovery of full function can be difficult s/p fracture-dislocation of the elbow.

Wrist Trauma

The scaphoid is the most commonly fractured bone in the wrist, typically a result of falling on an outstretched hand – scapholunate dislocation/instability and/or distal radius fracture can be associated. Pain upon palpation through the snuff-box warrants radiographic assessment with the "stretch or navicular" view required. A fractured hook of the hamate is less common and is associated with falls or impacts to the ulnar side of the wrist – a carpal tunnel view should be obtained along with the standard radiographs (Schaffer 1994; Resnik 2000; Daniels 2004). Keinböch's (lunate) and Preiser's (scaphoid) diseases are the end stage result of an undetected fracture that has led to avascular necrosis – a history of a fall onto an outstretched hand is the most common onset.

The identification of wrist instability is important regardless of the mechanism of onset; blunt trauma, trivial trauma or cumulative strain. Cerezal et. al. (2012) provides a good review of the emerging role of CT or MR arthrography in improving the diagnostic accuracy of these lesions – a growing recognition of the importance of dynamic radiographic assessment.

The Mayo classification for carpal instability identifies 4 general groups (Carlsen 2008), as follows:

1. Carpal instability dissociative (CID) – instability within a row.
2. Carpal instability nondissociative (CIND) – instability between rows.
3. Carpal instability complex (CIC) – includes combinations within and between rows.
4. Adaptive carpus – secondary malpositioning of the carpal bone(s).

On the ulnar side of the wrist the Palmer's classification of Triangular Fibrocartilage Complex (TFCC) lesions is the reference standard from which conservative verses surgical management is planned (Oneson 1996). Recently high resolution sonography has shown promise in adding to diagnostic accuracy (Keogh 2004). The Palmer classification is as follows:

Class 1: Traumatic
Central perforation
Ulnar avulsion (with and without styloid fracture)
Distal avulsion (from carpus)
Radial avulsion (with and without sigmoid notch fracture)

Class 2: Degenerative (Ulnar Impaction Syndrome)
TFCC wear
TFCC wear + lunate and/or ulnar head chondromalacia
TFCC perforation + lunate and/or ulnar head chondromalacia
TFCC perforation + lunate and/or ulnar head chondromalacia + lunotriquetral ligament perforation
TFCC perforation + lunate and/or ulnar head chondromalacia + lunotriquetral ligament perforation + ulnocarpal arthritis

There are many other upper limb traumatic injuries to consider but that are beyond the scope of this book because the focus is on cumulative and degenerative MSDs.

Considerations with Lower Limb Trauma

Athletic injuries, motor vehicle accidents and falls etc. are common causes of trauma to the lower limb. The possibility of fracture of the lower limb, particularly the hip or ankle increases significantly in the elderly (Baron 1996). Kaye and Jick (2004) reported that road collisions, dementia, use of corticosteroids, antipsychotics, antidepressants and hypnotic/sedative medications were all associated with an elevated risk for lower limb fracture. This is an important focus for MSD prevention, especially for the geriatric populations – a reason for the increased attention to balance and proprioceptive training programs. Barrett et. al (1999) reports the risk for fracture in a 65 year old by the age of 90 years is 16% for the hip, 9% for the distal forearm, 5% proximal humerus and 4% for the ankle – most of these associated with falls.

The knee joint is particularly vulnerable to both contact and non-contact traumatic injury. ACL injuries have received great attention with development of prevention programs that have evidence of efficacy (Hewett 1999; Mandelbaum 2005). These injuries tend to occur when the foot is planted with the knee at or close to extension and a valgus-collapse upon attempting rapid deceleration-acceleration (Boden 2000; Withrow 2006). Training programs that include a focus on developing good biomechanical technique, endurance, co-contraction of the hamstrings and quadriceps, balance and proprioception have proven effective (Ju 2010; Fujiya 2011; Kulas 2012). These same concepts apply to prevention of ankle sprains and fall-related injuries in general.

Ankle and foot injuries

Ankle sprains are a common injury in the general population with an incidence rate of 2.15 per 1000 person-years in the United States (Waterman 2010). Approximately half occur with athletic activities, and the incidence is highest between the ages of 15 – 19 years of age; but affect all age groups and frequently results in residual impairment and disability (Yeung 1994; Valderrabano 2006; Maliaropoulos 2009; Hiller 2011).

The possibility of fracture with lateral ankle injuries is the main red flag to proceeding with typical conservative treatment (Kerkhoffs 2012). This more likely with an eversion sprain, but can occur with the more common inversion injury.

The Ottawa Ankle Rules were developed to rule out fractures after acute injury (Bachmann 2003). These rules indicate that an ankle x-ray is required when there is pain in malleolar zone and any of the three following findings:

- Bony tenderness at the lateral malleolar zone A (from the tip of the lateral malleolus to include the lower 6 cm of posterior border of the fibula).
- Bony tenderness at the medial malleolar zone B (from the tip of the medial malleolus to the lower 6cm of the posterior border of the tibia).
- Inability to walk four weight bearing steps immediately after the injury and in the emergency room.

A foot x-ray is required if there is pain in the midfoot zone and any of the three following findings:

- Bone tenderness at navicular bone.
- Bone tenderness at base of 5th metatarsal.
- Inability to weight bear both immediately after the injury and in the emergency room.

References Chapter 9

Alyas F, Curtis M, Speed C, Saifuddin A, Connell D. MR Imaging appearances of acromioclavicular dislocation, Radiographics 28 (2): 463-79, 2008.

Appelboam A, Reuben AD, Benger JR, et. al. Elbow extension test to rule out elbow fracture: multicenter, prospective validation and observational study of diagnostic accuracy in adults and children. BMJ 2008; 337:a2428 (published 9 December 2008).

Bachmann LM, Kolb E, Koller MT, et. al. Accuracy of Ottawa ankle rules to exclude fractures of the ankle and mid-foot: systemic review. BMJ 326: 417, 2003.

Bagley LJ. Imaging of spinal trauma. Radiol Clin N Am 44: 1-12, 2006.

Baron JA, Karagas M, Barrett J, et. al. Basic epidemiology of fractures of the upper and lower limb among Americans over 65 years of age. Epidemiology 7 (6): 612-18, 1996.

Barrett JA, Baron JA, Karagas MR, Beach ML. Fracture risk in the US Medicare population. J Clin Epidemiology 52 (3): 243-49, 1999.

Berry GE, Adams S, Harris MB, et. al. Are plain radiographs of the spine necessary during evaluation after blunt trauma? Accuracy of screening torso computed tomography in thoracic/lumbar spine fracture diagnosis. J Trauma 59 (6): 1410-13, 2005.

Boden BP, Dean GS, Feagin JA, et. al. Mechanism of anterior cruciate ligament injury. Orthopedics 23: 573-78, 2000.

Buckwalter JA. Articular cartilage injuires. Clin Orthop Relat Res 402: 21-37, 2002.

Campbell SE, Phillips CD, Dubovsky E, et. al. The value of CT in determining potential instability of simple wedge-compression fractures of the lumbar spine. AJNR Am J Neuroradiol 16: 1385-92, 1995.

Carlsen BT, Shin AY. Wrist instability. Scand J Surg 97: 324-32, 2008.

Cerezal L, de Dios Berná-Mestre J, Canga A, et. al. MR and CT arthrography of the wrist. Semin Musculoskelet Radiol 16 (1): 27-41, 2012.

Cetik O, Uslu M, Ozsar BK. The relationship between Hill-Sachs lesion and recurrent anterior disolocation Acta Orthop Belg 73: 175-78, 2007.

Chamberlain CS, Crowley E, Vanderby R. The spatio-temporal dynamics of ligament healing. Wound Repair Regen. 2009; 17 (2): 206-215. Doi:10.1111/j.1524-475X.2009.00465.x.

Čičak N, Bilić, Delimar D. Hill-Sachs lesion in recurrent shoulder dislocation: sonographic detection. J Ultrasound Med 1&: 557-60, 1998.

Daniels JM, Zook EG, Lynch JM. Hand and wrist injuries: nonemergent evaluation. Am Fam Physician 69 (8): 1941-48, 2004.

Dearden C, Hughes D. Does the national emergency x-ray utilization study make a difference? Eur J Emerg Med 12: 278-81, 2005.

Dickinson G, Stiell IG, Schull M, et. al. Retrospective application of the NEXUS low-risk criteria for cervical spine radiography in Canadian emergency departments. Ann Emerg Med 43: 507-14, 2004.

Frush DP. Review of radiation issues for computed tomography. Semin Ultrasound CT MR 25: 15-24, 2004.

Fujiya H, Kousa P, Fleming BC, et. al. Effect of muscle loads and torque applied to the tibia on the strain behavior of the anterior cruciate ligament: an in vitro investigation. Clinical Biomechanics 26: 1005-11, 2011.

Geeraerts T, Chhor V, Cheisson G, et. al. Clinical review: initial management of blunt pelvic trauma patients with haemodynamic instability. Critical Care 2007, 11:204 (doi:10.1186/cc5157) available online:http://ccforum.com/content/11/1/204

Godefroy D, Rousselin B, Sarazin L. Imaging of traumatic injuries of the elbow [Article in

French]. J Radiol 2007 May; 88(5Pt2): 734-40.

Guillamondegui OD, Pryor JP, Gracias VH, Gupta R, Reilly PM, Schwab CW. Pelvic radiography in blunt trauma resuscitation: a diminishing role. J Trauma 53 (6): 1043-7, 2002.

Heffernan DS, Schermer CR, Lu SW. What defines a distracting injury in cervical spine assessment? J Trauma Injury Infect Crit Care 59: 1396-99, 2005.

Herzog C, Ahle H, Mack MG, et. al. Traumatic injuires of the pelvis and thoracic and lumbar spine: does thin-slice multidetector-row CT increase diagnostic accuracy? Eur Radiol 14: 1751-60, 2004.

Hewett TE, Lindenfeld TN, Riccobene JV, et. al. The effect of neuromuscular training on the incidence of knee injury in female athletes: a propspective study. Am J Spts Med 27: 699-706, 1999.

Hiller CE, Nightingale EJ, Lin CW, et. al. Characteristics of people with recurrent ankle sprains: a systematic review with meta-analysis. Br J Sports Med 45 (8): 660-72, 2011.

Ju YY, Wang CW, Cheng HYK. Effects of fatiguing movement versus passive repetitive movement on knee proprioception. Clinical Biomechanics 25: 708-12, 2010.

Kulas AS, Hortobágyi T, DeVita P. Trunk position modulates anterior cruciate ligament forces and strains during a single-leg squat. Clinical Biomechanics 27: 16 – 21, 2012.

Mandelbaum BR, Silvers HJ, Watanabe D, et. al. Effectiveness of a neuromuscular and proprioceptive training program in preventing anterior cruciate ligament injuiries in female athletes.: two year follow up. Am J Spts Med 33: 1003-10, 2005.

Hoffman JR, Schriger DL, Mower W, et.al. Low-risk criteria for cervical spine radiography in blunt trauma: a prospective study. Ann Emerg Med 21: 1454-60, 1992.

Hoffman JR. Validity of a set of clinical criteria to rule out injury to the cervical spine in patients with blunt trauma. NEJM 343: 94-99, 2000.

Hoffman JR, Mower WR, Wolfson AB, et. al. Validity of a set of clinical criteria to rule out injury to the cervical spine in patients with blunt trauma. National Emergency X-Radiography Utilization Study Group N Engl J Med 343 (1): 94-9, 2000.

Holmes JF, Akkinepalli R. Computed tomography versus plain radiography to screen cervical spine injury: a meta-analysis. J Trauma Injury Infect Crit Care 58: 902-5, 2005.

Hsu SL, Liang R, Woo SLY. Functional tissue engineering of ligament healing. Sports Medicine, Arthroscopy, Rehabilitation, Therapy & Technology 2010, 2:12 http://www.smarttjournal .com/content/2/1/12

Kalfas IH Principles of bone healing. Neurosurg Focus 10 (4): 1 – 10 (Article 1), 2001.

Kaye JA, Jick H. Epidemiology of lower limb fractures in general practice in the United Kingdom. Injury Prevention 2004; 10: 368-374. doi: 10.1136/ip.2004.005843.

Keogh CF, Wong AD, Wells NJ, Barbarie JE, Cooperberg PL. High-resolution sonography of the triangular fibrocartilage: initial experience and correlation with MRI and arthroscopic findings. AJR 182:333 – 36, 2004.

Keramaris NC, Calori GM, Nikolaou VS, Schemitsch EH, Giannoudis PV. Fracture vascularity and bone healing: a systematic review of the role of VEGF. Injury 39 (Suppl 2): S45-57, 2008.

Kerkhoffs GM, van den Bekerom M, Elders LAM, et. al. Diagnosis, treatment and prevention of ankle sprains: an evidence-based clinical guideline. Br J Sports Med 46: 854-60, 2012.

Kerr D, Bradshaw L, Kelly AM. Implementaiton of the Canadian C-spine rule reduces cervical spine x-ray rate for alert patients with potential neck injury. J Emerg Med 28: 127-31, 2005.

Kessel B, Sevi R, Jeroukhimov I, et. al. Is routine portable pelvic x-ray in stable multiple trauma patients always justified in a high technology era? Injury 38 (5): 559-63, 2007.

Kuhn MA, Ross G. Acute elbow dislocations. Orth Clinic North Am 39 (2): 155-61, 2008.

Laffosse JM, Reina N, Tricoire JL, Chiron P, Puget J. Variants of the shoulder side impact syndrome: the posterior sternoclavicular dislocation. Orthop Traum Surg Res 96 (7): 816-20, 2010.

Lampraikis A, Vlasis K, Siampou E, Grammatikopoulos I, Louis C. Can elbow-extension test be used as an alternative to radiographs in primary care? Eur J Gen Pract 13 (4): 221-24, 2007.

Hewett TE, Lindenfeld TN, Riccobene JV, et. al. The effect of neuromuscular training on the incidence of knee injury in female athletes: a propspective study. Am J Spts Med 27: 699-706, 1999.

Malliaropoulos N, Ntessalen M, Papacostas E, Longo UG, Maffulli N. Reinjury after acute lateral ankle sprains in elite track and field athletes. Am J Sports Med 37 (9): 1755-61, 2009.

Mandelbaum BR, Silvers HJ, Watanabe D, et. al. Effectiveness of a neuromuscular and proprioceptive training program in preventing anterior cruciate ligament injuiries in female athletes.: two year follow up. Am J Spts Med 33: 1003-10, 2005.

Mihoefer K, McAdams TR, Scopp JM, Mandelbaum BR. Emerging options for treatment of articular cartilage injury in the athlete. Clin Sports Med 28 (1): 25-40, 2009.

Nemec U, Oberleithner G, Nemec SF, et. al. MRI versus radiography of acromioclavicular joint dislocation. AJR Am J Roentgenol 197 (4): 968-73, 2011.

Nordin M, Carragee EJ, Hogg-Johnson S, et. al. Assessment of neck pain and associated disorders: results of the bone and joint decade 2000-2010 task force on neck pain and its associated disorders. Spine 33 (4S): S101-122, 2008.

Oneson SR, Scales LM, Timins ME, Erickson SJ, Chamoy L. MR imaging interpretation of the Palmer classification of triangular fibrocartilage complex lesions. Radiographics 16 (1): 97 – 106, 1996.

Panacek EA, Mover WR, Holmes JF, et. al. Test performance of the individual NEXUS low-risk clinical screening criteria for cervical spine injury. Ann Emerg Med 38: 22 – 25, 2001.

Pollack CV Jr., Hendey GW, Martin DR, et. al. Use of flexion-extension radiographs of the cervical spine in blunt trauma. Ann Emerg Med 38: 8 – 11, 2001.

Resnik CS. Wrist and hand injuries. Semin Musculoskelet Radiol 4: 193-204, 2000.

Roos JE, Hilfiker P, Platz A, et. al. MDCT in emergency radiology: is a standardized chest of abdominal protocol sufficient for evaluation of the thoracic and lumbar spine trauma. Am J Roentgenol 183: 959-68, 2004.

Rowley G, Fielding K. Reliability and accuracy of the Glasgow Coma Scale with experienced and inexperienced users. Lancet 337: 535-38, 1991.

Sans N, Railhac JJ. Elbow: plain radiographs. J Radiol May 2008; 89(5 Pt 2):633-38, quiz 639.

Sasyniuk TM, Mohtadi NGH, Hollinshead RM, Russell ML, Fick GH. The inter-rater reliability of shoulder arthroscopy. J Arthroscopic Rel Surg 23 (9): 971-77, 2007.

Schaffer TC. Common hand fractures in family practice. Arch Fam Med 3: 982-87, 1994.

Sharma P, Maffulli N. Biology of tendon injury: healing, modeling and remodeling. J Musculoskelet Neuronal Interact 6 (2): 181-90, 2006.

Sheridan R, Peralta R, Rhea J, et. al. Reformatted visceral protocol helical computed tomographic scanning allows conventional radiographs of the thoracic and lumbar spine to be eliminated in the evaluation of blunt trauma patients. J Trauma 55: 665-69, 2003.

Spitzer WO, Skovron ML, Salmi LR, Cassidy JD, et al. Scientific monograph of the Quebec task force on whiplash-associated disorders: redefining 'whiplash' and its management. Spine 20 (8S), 1995.

Stiell I, McKnight R, Schull M, et. al. The Canadian C-spine rules versus the NEXUS low-risk criteria in patients with trauma. N Engl J Med 349: 2510-18, 2003.

Steill I, Wells GA, Vandemheem K. The Canadian C-spine rule for radiography in alert and stable trauma patients. JAMA 286: 1841-48, 2001.

Teasdale G, Jennett B. Assessment of coma and impaired consciousness. Lancet 304: 81-84, 1974

Teasdale G, Jennett B. Assessment and prognosis of coma after head injury. Acta Neurochir 34: 45-55, 1976.

Teasdale G, Kril-Jones R, van der Sande J. Observer variability in assessing impaired consciousness and coma. J Neurol Neurosurg Psychiatry 41: 603-10, 1978.

Towler DA. The osteogenic-angiogenic interface: novel insights into the biology of bone formation and fracture repair. Curr Osteoporos Rep 6 (2): 67-71, 2008.

Valderrabano V, Hintermann B, Horisberger M, Fung TS. Ligamentous posttraumatic ankle osteoarthritis. Am J Sports Med 34 (4): 612-20, 2006

Waterman BR, Owens BD, Davey S, Zacchilli MA, Belmont PJ. The epidemiology of ankle sprains in the United States. JBJS 92A (13): 2279-84, 2010 (a).

Waterman BR, Belmont PJ, Cameron KL, DeBerardino TM, Owens BD. Epidemiology of ankle sprain at the United States military academy. Am J Sports Med 38 (4): 797-803, 2010 (b).

Watura R, Cobby M, Taylor J. Multislice CT in imaging of trauma of the spine, pelvis and complex foot injuries. Br J Radiol 77: 46-63, 2004.

Withrow TJ, Huston LJ, Wojtys EM, Ashton-Miller JA. The effect of an impulsive knee valgus moment on in vitro relative ACL strain during a simulated jump landing. Clinical Biomechanics 21: 977-83, 2006.

Yeung MS, Kai-Ming C, So CH, Yuan WY. An epidemiological survey on ankle sprain. Br J Sp Med 28 (2): 112-16, 1994.

10 CAUTIONS & CONTRAINDICATIONS

The identification of patients with contraindications to physical therapy treatment, and those who have risk factors that require special attention and consideration is a critical component of quality healthcare and independent clinical practice. Over the past 10 – 20 years contraindications have become associated with the term 'red flags', and cautions with the term 'yellow flags'. This chapter adopts this terminology to distinguish these two groups. Red flags require suspension of any treatment and immediate referral and/or consultation with the patient's medical physician. Yellow flags require communication and coordination with the medical physician, special attention when implementing a treatment plan, and the possibility of suspending treatment until further work-up or evaluation has been completed.

In our system there is continuous assessment for red or yellow flags. This starts with the preliminary information provided by the patient (i.e. patient information form, pre-questionnaires etc.) and any diagnostic or clinical information provided by a referring physician. The next point of assessment is during the history and physical examination process; the identification, characteristics and behavior of the patient's symptoms and signs. This is followed by the ongoing evaluation of the patient's response to treatment during the course of their care.

Thankfully serious pathologies mimicking an activity-related MSD are rare. Greenhalgh and Selfe (2006) identify the incidence to be approximately 1% of patients seeking treatment for back or neck pain; Bogduk (2002) indicates that the risk for encountering a 'red flag' disorder or disease including cancer, in a patient presenting with a low back pain problem is < 1%. The APTA Manipulation Task Force (2004) states that the risk of cauda equina syndrome from lumbar manipulation is estimated to be on the order of 1 in 100 million manipulations – a miniscule risk, especially when compared to potential complication or death attributable to the incorrect administration of medications. Regardless of how small the risk, we need to be meticulous in our clinical processes and diligently on guard for the patient's well-being.

Contraindications ('Red Flags'):

The most common red flags for activity-related musculoskeletal disorders relate to injury as a result of trauma, previously undiagnosed disease, a recurrence or progression of a disease, or the progression of an MSD to include signs and symptoms that are unsuitable for physical therapy and require immediate medical attention (e.g. cauda equina syndrome, spondylotic myelopathy, VBI etc.).

1.   **S/P Trauma** – in my experience this is the most prevalent contraindication encountered in musculoskeletal care. This includes previously undetected fracture, subluxation, dislocation and/or instability. Any time the patient identifies a significant external force as the cause for the onset of their symptoms this needs to be considered, even if they have had previous imaging or diagnostic work-up – the results may have been false negative. This was covered in a separate chapter – be familiar with the most reliable and validated diagnostic tools and always give precedence to the patient's clinical presentation when previous studies are unremarkable.

2.   **Undiagnosed disease** – the medical system is generally good at screening most of these patients, but it is by no means perfect. The most significant contraindications include malignancies, systemic inflammatory diseases, osteogenic diseases, benign tumors, congenital anomalies, endocrine/metabolic disorders, neurologic and vascular diseases. These diseases or disorders could have been the cause of the symptoms from the start, or it is possible that a patient coincidentally has an onset during the course of physical therapy treatment.

A common factor with this group of patients is a lack of mechanical behavior of their signs and symptoms, plus atypical clinical findings for an activity-related MSD. A good history-taker and objective examiner usually picks up on this quickly. Know your populations at risk; i.e. age, gender, ethnicity, occupation and other demographic considerations that affect vulnerability. John Mennell, MD taught physical therapists in 1970-80s to have an oral thermometer in their clinic because any patient presenting with musculoskeletal pain and a fever is a contraindication until worked-up by the medical physician.

3. Recurrence or progression of a disease – it is always possible that a recurrence or the sequellae of a disease has been mistaken for a MSD. The identification process is the same as with undiagnosed disease with the one major exception; there was a previous or current history that should have immediately put you on guard. Cancer is a classic example of this; when the patient is > 50 years of age and has a previous history of cancer the likelihood of the diagnosis increases significantly (Henscke 2007; 2009).

4. Progression of an activity-related MSD – examples of this include; a lumbar disc disorder progressing into a large central herniation causing compression of the S3,4 roots; a cervical or thoracic disc disorder progressing into a spondylotic myelopathy; a mechanical neck disorder beginning to exhibit signs and symptoms of vertebra-basilar artery insufficiency (VBI) etc.

We need to be on guard – as a general rule start treatment conservatively with stage 3 disorders, opting to control aggravating factors and the symptoms before directly attempting to eliminate signs.

Sizer et. al. (2007) identifies 3 categories when screening patients with spine pain disorders for red flags (see table 10-1). This is a good general review, plus it provides a ranking of priority for immediate medical attention.

Additionally, Bogduk (2002;2006) provides a checklist for quick screening of patients with low back and neck pain disorders; Underwood (2009) attempts to put the screening process into a perspective; and Ross and Boissonnault (2010) present an excellent editorial on the subject.

Table 10-1: Sizer's 3 categories when screening patients for red flags with spine pain disorders.		
Category 1: Factors that require immediate medical attention	**Category 2: Factors that require subjective questioning and precautionary examination and treatment procedures**	**Category 3: Factors that require further physical testing and differentiation analysis**
Blood in sputum	Age > 50 years	Abnormal reflexes
Loss of consciousness or altered mental state	Clonus (could be a past CNS disorder)	Bilateral or unilateral radiculopathy or
Neurologic deficit not explained by mono-radiculopathy	Fever	paresthesias
	Elevated sedimentation rate	Unexplained referred
	Gait deficits	pain
Numbness or paresthesias in perianal region	History of a disorder with predilection for infection or hemorrhage	Unexplained significant upper or
Pathological changes in bowel and bladder	History of cancer	lower limb weakness
	Impairment precipitated by recent trauma	
Patterns of symptoms not compatible with mechanical pain (on physical exam)	Long-term corticosteroid use	
	Long-term workers' compensation	
Progressive neurologic deficit	Non-healing sores or wounds	
Pulsatile abdominal masses	Recent history of unexplained weight loss	
	Writhing pain	

Cautions ('Yellow Flags'):

The presence of yellow flags is far more common in clinical practice. These cautions do not necessarily preclude physical therapy treatment; rather they require recognition of the need for special considerations in treatment planning and assessment of patient response. This includes the possibility that treatment should be suspended pending further medical evaluation and/or help from another discipline to address relevant issues. A therapist that routinely customizes their treatment plans to the needs of the individual patient segues to this strategy easily. Yellow flags fall into several categories that include; psychosocial findings, medications and possible side effects (iatrogenic factors), co-morbidities and others.

Psychosocial Factors

We have stressed the importance of recognizing the potential adverse effects of psychosocial issues. The Accident Compensation Commission in New Zealand released a report addressing these yellow flags in 1997, providing clinicians with evidenced-based guidelines. These included: adverse attitudes and beliefs, behaviors, compensation issues, diagnosis and treatment, emotions, family and work issues (see table 10-2). This is a good overview.

Factor	Description
Table 10-2: Yellow flags taken from the NZ acute LBP guide (ACC 1997): these are psychosocial, clinical and occupational factors that can adversely impact a patient's response to treatment and are predisposing to disability.	
Attitudes and Beliefs	• Belief that pain is harmful or disabling resulting in fear-avoidance behavior. • Belief that all pain must be abolished before attempting to RTW or normal activity. • Catastrophizing, thinking the worst, misinterpreting bodily symptoms. • Belief that pain is uncontrollable. • Passive attitude to rehabilitation.
Behaviors	• Use of extended rest, disproportionate 'downtime'. • Reduced activity level with significant withdrawal from activities of daily living. • Irregular participation or poor compliance with physical exercise, tendency for activities to be in a 'boom-bust' cycle. • Avoidance of normal activity and progressive substitution of lifestyle away from productive activity. • Report of extremely high intensity of pain; e.g. above 10 on a 0-10 VAS. • Excessive reliance on use of aids or appliances. • Sleep quality reduced since onset of pain. • High intake of alcohol and other substances (possibly as self-medication), with an increase since onset of back pain. • Smoking.
Compensation Issues	• Lack of financial incentive to RTW. • Delay in assessing income support and treatment cost, disputes over eligibility. • History of claim(s) due to other injuries or pain problems. • History of extended time off work due to injury or other pain problem (e.g. > 12 wks.). • History of previous back pain with previous claim(s) and time off work. • Previous experience of ineffective case management (e.g. absence of interest, perception of being treated punitively).
Diagnosis and Treatment	• Health professionals sanctioning disability, not providing interventions that will improve function. • Experience of conflicting diagnoses or explanation for back pain resulting in confusion. • Diagnostic language leading to catastrophizing and fear (e.g. fear of ending up in a wheelchair). • Dissatisfaction of back pain by health professional producing dependency on treatments, and continuation of passive treatment. • Number of times visited health professional in last year (excluding the present episode of back pain). • Expectation of a 'techno-fix'; e.g. requests to treat as if body were a machine. • Lack of satisfaction with previous treatment for back pain. • Advice to withdraw from job. <div align="right">Continued next page</div>

Emotions	• Fear of increased pain with activity or work. • Depression (especially long-term low mood), loss of sense of enjoyment. • More irritable than usual. • Anxiety about and heightened awareness of body sensations includes sympathetic nervous system arousal. • Feeling under stress and unable to maintain control. • Presence of social anxiety or disinterest in social activity. • Feeling useless and not needed.
Family	• Over-protective partner/spouse, emphasizing fear of harm or encouraging catastrophizing (usually well intentioned). • Solicitous behavior from spouse (e.g. taking over tasks). • Socially punitive responses from spouse (e.g. ignoring, expressing frustration). • Extent to which family members support any attempt to RTW. • Lack of support person to talk to about problems.
Work	• History of manual work, notably from the following occupational groups: fishing, forestry and farming workers; construction, including carpenters and builders; nurses, trunk drivers, laborers. • Work history including patterns of frequent job changes, experiencing stress at work, job dissatisfaction, and poor relationships with peers or supervisors, lack of vocational direction. • Belief that work is harmful; that it will do damage or be dangerous. • Unsupportive or unhappy current work environment. • Low educational background, low socioeconomic status. • Job involves significant bio-mechanical demands, such as lifting, manual handling heavy items, extended sitting, extended standing, driving, vibration, maintenance of constrained or sustained postures, inflexible work schedule preventing appropriate breaks. • Job involves shift work or working unsociable hours. • Minimal availability of selected duties and graduated RTW pathways, with unsatisfactory implementation of these. • Negative experience of workplace management of back pain (e.g. absence of a reporting system, discouragement to report, punitive response from supervisors and managers). • Absence of interest from employer.

Medication Side Effects

Pharmaceutical manufacturing is a big business, there are many people taking prescription medications, and many have possible side effects that could mimic or affect a musculoskeletal problem (see table below). I recommend that you become familiar with potential side-effects by routinely researching information about the medications your patients are taking until you are familiar. When in doubt discuss with the patient's family physician or the prescribing physician – keep in mind that the side effects may be from the combination of medications taken rather than any particular medication, and dose matters.

The incorrect prescription of medication is a major source of medical error – this is a significant and growing problem. In the United States medical error in hospitals results in 44,000 – 98,000 unnecessary deaths each year and 1,000,000 excess injuries (Weingart 2000). The CDC (2011) reports that three out of every four prescription drug overdoses are caused by painkillers, a 300% increase since 1999, representing 14,800 overdose deaths in 2008.

The fact that there are more medications on the market, the ubiquity of drug advertisements through mass media, and the fact that more people are taking more medications renders a significant concern for all healthcare practitioners (see table 10-3). In addition, the greater availability of nonprescription (alternative) medications and supplements requires continual diligence for the patient's well-being. Thank goodness for the internet and the search engines that render this task less difficult.

Table 10-3: Medical Expenditure Panel Survey: Prescribed Drug Estimates in the United States: 2005. Top 25 prescribed drugs by total expenditures, total purchases and reported possible side-effects that could be mistaken for musculoskeletal disorder and/or represent a caution for physical therapy. (www.meps.ahrq.gov/mepsweb)

Rx Drug	Action	Total Expenditure	Tot. # Persons	Possible Musculoskeletal Side-effects & Cautions for PT
Lipitor	Cholesterol lowering	9,311,420,518	15,103,266	Muscle pain, tenderness, weakness
Zocor	Cholesterol lowering	5,661,620,311	7,389,886	Muscle pain, tenderness, weakness
Procrit	Produce red blood cells	5,405,531,976	150,641	Risk to develop DVT, esp. perisurgery
Nexium	Anti-acid	4,411,844,401	5,198,113	Headache
Advair	Anti-inflammatory/ asthma	3,572,482,585	5,477,687	Headache + general concerns for steroids
Prevacid	Anti-acid	3,542,363,243	5,652,574	Headache
Plavix	Anti-coagulant	3,496,506,916	4,278,831	Sudden headache (+/-confusion), weakness (esp. one side of body), chest/arm pain + uncontrolled bleeding
Zoloft	Anti-depressant	2,972,819,923	5,460,661	Seizure, loss balance/co-ordination, drowsiness, dizziness, weakness.
Lisinopril	Anti-hypertension	2,705,815,749	9,883,880	Light-headed, fainting, aching, drowsiness, dizziness, weakness.
Norvasc	Anti-hypertension/angina	2,593,782,341	6,467,478	Swelling ankles/feet, dizziness/fainting, fatigue/tiredness, headache.

Singulair	Anti-asthma	2,490,396,925	5,354,568	Severe tingling, numbness, pain, muscle weakness, dizziness, headache, mouth pain.
Atenolol	Anti-hyper-tension /angina (Beta-blocker)	2,146,636,611	7,964,126	Light-headed/fainting, swelling ankles/feet, dizziness, fatigue/tiredness.
Protonix	Anti-acid	2,129,191,014	3,754,719	Headache
Metformin	Anti-diabetic	2,057,425,117	6,182,782	Shortness of breath, swelling, body aches, headache, muscle pain, weakness.
Diovan	Anti-hypertension/CHF	2,033,266,638	4,435,404	Light-headed, fainting, aching, drowsiness, seizure, muscle pain/weakness, joint pain, headache, dizziness, insomnia.
Fosamax	Anti-osteoporosis	1,984,138,720	4,146,012	chest pain, dysphagia, pain/burning ribs or back, severe joint/bone/muscle pain, jaw pain, numbness, swelling, swelling, back pain, dizziness, weakness, headache.
Lexapro	Anti-depressant	1,953,960,221	4,927,642	Seizure, tremors, shivering, muscle stiffness or twitching, loss balance/co-ordination, headache, drowsiness, dizziness, restless.
Effexor	Anti-depressant	1,938,322,170	3,188,639	Severe headache, blurred vision, loss of coordination, fainting, seizure, weakness, easy bruising or bleeding, drowsiness, dizziness, nervousness.
Toprol	Anti-hypertension/angina (Beta-blocker)	1,796,056,106	6,396,135	Light-headed/fainting, swelling ankles/feet, dizziness, fatigue/tiredness.
Allegra	Anti-histamine	1,770,137,524	6,726,634	Nausea, drowsiness, tired feeling, headache, muscle or back pain.
Actos	Anti-diabetic	1,753,091,037	2,026,908	Short of breath, swelling, blurred vision, easy bruising or bleeding, weakness, headache, muscle pain.
Celebrex	NSAID	1,689,732,614	3,756,771	Weakness, shortness of breath, slurred speech, problems with vision or balance, swelling, headache with blistering, peeling, and red skin rash, bruising, severe tingling, numbness, pain, muscle weakness, dizziness, tinnitus.
Zyprexa	Anti-psychotic	1,628,418,784	703,668	Stiff muscles, jerky/uncontrolled muscle movements, sudden numbness or weakness (esp. one side of the body), sudden headache, confusion, problems with vision, speech, or balance, weakness, light-headed/fainting, dizziness, drowsiness, swelling, back pain.
Pravachol	Cholesterol Lowering	1,611,158,993	2,197,539	Muscle pain/tenderness, weakness, tired feeling, headache, dizziness, skin rash, general pain.
Zyrtec	Anti-histamine	1,549,766,230	6,480,214	Fatigue, dizziness, headaches.

Comorbidities

The presence of coexisting diseases, disorders or other relevant factors above and beyond the patient's MSD is a growing concern and source for caution in treatment planning. The most common comorbidities encountered are diabetes, cardiovascular and/or lung disease, osteoporosis and obesity – but the list of possibilities is almost endless. According to Booth (2000) we are currently losing the war against chronic diseases – the good news is that we can win this war through the application of exercise biology.

There are also orthopaedic comorbidities, including those resulting from failed or partially effective surgical treatment (Deyo 2004). For example, spine surgery rates in the US are 40% greater than any other country and five times higher than the UK (Cherkin 1994); the rates of lumbar fusion increased 220% from 1996 to 2001 (Deyo 2005); 433% for cervical fusion and 356% for lumbar fusion between 1997 and 2003 (Cowan 2006). Musculoskeletal comorbidities also include patients with more than one active musculoskeletal injury – this is most likely in patients with a traumatic onset to their problem (Spitzer 1995).

In the case of assessing and treating patients with comorbidities the recovery is often slower, treatment procedures may require modifications, and you need to pay attention for adverse changes related to the comorbidities. In some cases you may need to lower the functional goals and expectations to an appropriate level and/or you may need to work more closely with the patient's medical practitioner.

Other Factors

Simply the failure to recover from an MSD in a reasonable amount of time with well executed, active and evidenced based care is a yellow flag. This was an important component of the management guidelines of the 'Quebec Task Force Report' for activity-related spinal disorders (Spitzer 1987). A critical pathway strategy was divided into three timeframes with the intent of getting the patient (appropriately) back to normal work activities in the shortest possible time. The first point of complete reassessment was recommended between weeks 4 - 7, as most back and pain patients should have recovered and return to work/activity. The idea was to discover why the patient isn't responding through diagnostic testing and/or specialist consultation. Findings should guide appropriate adjustments to the treatment plan and most should recover. Should this new strategy be unsuccessful the next point of complete reassessment should occur at > 3 months. The patient's condition has become chronic, a specific structural or medical diagnosis has been ruled-out, so now a multidisciplinary assessment team is suggested (i.e. remember this is for workers unable to RTW). Often there are overlapping yellow flag factors that are relevant.

Comments

Over the years Jean and I have referred dozens of our patients back to their medical physician because we suspected something seriously wrong or not of a mechanical, activity-related source. The eventual diagnoses that were mimicking a MSD have included: ovarian cystic disease/endometriosis, lung cancer with metastasis to the spine, stress fractures (multiple sites), fracture-dislocation cervical spine, osteosarcoma of the proximal femur, ankylosing spondylitis, subclavian artery steal syndrome, neurofibromatosis, peripheral vascular disease, adverse reaction to statin drugs, tethered cord syndrome and more. When the patient's signs and symptoms do not behave mechanically and/or the patient does not seem well, refer them to their medical physician for evaluation. Batavia (2006) has published a textbook that provides a comprehensive coverage of contraindications for physical rehabilitation - "primum non nocere".

In regards to yellow flags, it appears that clinical practice has become more complex on many fronts over the past 10 – 20 years. Navigating the insurance system to provide care to patients and be appropriately reimbursed is certainly more complex than it used to be. Patients are coming to therapy with more diagnoses, taking more medications, more people are having elective surgeries and chronic illnesses are on the rise. This exemplifies the need for prevention oriented healthcare – but in the meantime the patient with yellow flags remains a challenge. Look at these clinical situations as an opportunity to learn, and remain focused on function and long-term health. The DRS 5 core elements apply once the various 'yellow flag' factors have been identified and addressed.

References Chapter 10

ACC and the National Health Committee (1997). New Zealand acute low back pain guide. Ministry of Health & Accident Rehabilitation and Compensation Insurance Corporation. Wellington, New Zealand

APTA Manipulation Task Force Manipulation Education Manual: For Physical Therapist Professional Degree Programs. APTA, April 2004.

Batavia M. Contraindications in Physical Rehabilitation: Doing No Harm. St. Louis, MO, Saunders Elsevier, 2006.

Bogduk N, McGuirk B. Pain Research and Clinical Management; Vol. 13: Medical Management of Acute and Chronic Low Back Pain. An Evidence-based Approach. Elsevier, Amsterdam, 2002.

Bogduk N, McGuirk B. Pain Research and Clinical Management: Pain Research and Clinical Management of Acute and Chronic Neck Pain. An Evidence-based Approach. Edinburgh, Elsevier, 2006.

Booth FW, Gordon SE, Carlson CJ, Hamilton MT. Waging war on modern chronic diseases: primary prevention through exercise biology. Journal Applied Physiology 88: 774-87, 2000.

CDC. Vital Signs: overdoses of prescription opioid pain relievers – United States, 1999 – 2008. MMWR 2011; 60: 1-6.

Cherkin DC, Deyo R, Loeser JD, et al. An international comparison of back surgery rates. Spine 11 (10):1201–6, 1994.

Cowan JA Jr, Dimick JB, Wainess R, Upchurch GR Jr, Chandler WF, La Marca F. Changes in the utilization of spinal fusion in the United States. Neurosurgery 59 (1):15-20, 2006.

Deyo RA, Nachemson A, Mirza SK. Spinal-fusion surgery-the case for restraint. NEJM 350 (7): 722-26, 2004.

Deyo RA, Gray DT, Kreuter W, Mirza S, Martin BI. United States trends in lumbar fusion surgery for degenerative conditions. Spine 30 (12):1441-1445, 2005.

Greenhalgh S, Selfe J. Red Flags: A Guide to Identifying Serious Pathology of the Spine. Edinburgh, Churchill Livingstone, 2006.

Henschke N, Maher CG, Refshauge KM. Screening for malignancy in low back pain patients: a systematic review. Eur Spine J 16:1673–1679, 2007.

Henschke N, Maher CG, Refshauge KM, et al. Prevalence of and Screening for Serious Spinal Pathology in Patients Presenting to Primary Care Settings With Acute Low Back Pain. Arthritis Rheumatism. 60 (10):3072-80, 2009.

Medical Expenditure Panel Survey: Prescribed Drug Estimates in the United States: 2005. (www.meps.ahrq.gov/mepsweb)

Nordin M, Carragee EJ, Hogg-Johnson S, et. al. Assessment of neck pain and associated disorders: results of the bone and joint decade 2000-2010 task force on neck pain and its associated disorders. Spine 33 (4S): S101-122, 2008.

Ross MD, Boissonnault WG. Red flags: to screen or not to screen? JOSPT 40 (11): 682-84, 2010.

Spitzer WO, Skovron ML, Salmi LR, Cassidy JD, et al. Scientific monograph of the Quebec task force on whiplash-associated disorders: redefining 'whiplash' and its management. Spine 20 (8S), 1995.

Underwood M. Diagnosing acute nonspecific low back pain: time to lower the red flags? Arthritis Care Research 60 (10): 2855-57, 2009.

Weingart SN, Willson RM, Gibberd RW, Harrison B. Epidemiology of medical error. BMJ2000; 320; 774-77 doi:10.1136/bmj.320.7237.774.

11 TREATMENT STRATEGIES, REASSESSMENT & PROBLEM-SOLVING

Treatment is the implementation of a plan that guides the patient back to their normal musculoskeletal status and function. The characteristics of musculoskeletal disorders are clinically expressed as symptoms, signs, interference with normal activities of daily living (ADL), and the patient's cognitive, psychological and emotional response to the problem. The efficacy of treatment is measured by the ability to eliminate or control these signs and symptoms, and remove their interference with the patient's normal ADL. This is how we challenge ourselves to prove the applied truth of our clinical and therapeutic conclusions, clinical models and therapeutic strategies. This challenge is accepted and measured one patient at a time.

However, the most important measure of the success of treatment begins after discharge and includes; prevention of recurrence or progression of the same disorder, the maintenance of activity tolerance and physical performance capability, and evidence of musculoskeletal self-efficacy. The DRS treatment strategies are designed to promote this long-term effect by customizing the plan to the unique characteristics of the individual patient's problem and training them to actively participate in their recovery; i.e. encouraging musculoskeletal self-efficacy. Self-efficacy is defined as; a "resilient self-belief system in the face of obstacles" (Bandura 1989; Nicholas 2007).

There are many ways to implement a successful treatment plan; however there are common factors to successful treatment identified by Hubble (1999):

The client/extratherapeutic factors – this refers to the patient's inherent strengths, support factors and their general life circumstances. This has been found to account for up to 40 % of outcome variance.

Relationship factors: this refers to the empathy, warmth, acceptance, mutual affirmation etc. experienced by the therapeutic bond/rapport established between the patient and caregiver. This has been found to account for up to 30 % of outcome variance.

Placebo, hope and expectancy factors: this refers to credibility, belief, restorative power of procedures and rituals etc. - the effect of knowing that something professional is being done and the confidence that it will help (i.e. positive placebo). This has been found to account for up to 15 % of the outcome variance.

Model/technique factors: this refers to the specific school of thought, the beliefs and procedures used in that system. This has been found to account for up to 15 % of the outcome variance. Possibly one of the reasons why it has been so difficult to prove that one system of treatment is clearly superior to others in MSD efficacy studies.

This research was conducted for psychotherapy, but it has applicability to the physical therapy treatment of spine pain and cumulative strain disorders and disability. There is face-validity as most MSDs are lifestyle-generated along with the abundance of evidence that psychosocial factors have a significant impact on treatment outcomes.

Six Treatment Strategies

In our system the patient is sent off after the initial visit with one of six treatment plans (see table 11-1). This range of strategies enables us to successfully treat the widest cross-section of MSDs possible.

1.   **Anti-inflammatory** - the goal in this strategy is to turn the pain from constant and easily exacerbated to intermittent and stable. This is achieved through instruction and training of the patient in the most effective mid-range (resting) positions for the tissues/structures involved in the disorder. Treatment can include the use of anti-inflammatory modalities (ice, phono and iontophoresis, electric stimulation etc.) in conjunction with medications prescribed by the medical doctor. However, the focus is on physical/biomechanical methods to gain control of aggravating factors. The patient is advised to

remain active to tolerance. Once the condition is stable and the symptoms begin to behave with a mechanical nociceptive pattern, the treatment strategy progresses to posture-ergonomic, remodeling, reduction or stabilization guidelines. In other words, the anti-inflammatory strategy is always a transitional one.

2.   Posture/ergonomic – this treatment plan centers on educating and training the patient in self-management skills. Stage I disorders always fall into this treatment plan. Therefore, how early you are intervening in the development of a disorder influences the frequency of using this treatment plan as the sole method of intervention. You man also chose to use this treatment plan for Stage II & III disorders if you want to be more conservative in your approach, provided there is mechanical behavior of the RSSx. This plan is in the rapid response grouping.

Postural/ergonomic training and the development of an individualized TTFB® system is the foundation of the Duffy-Rath System© and is included as a component of all interventions (modified according to response grouping). The following are the main components of the posture-ergonomic strategy: 1) Postural Retraining, 2) Body Mechanic Retraining, 3) Strategic Micro-pauses, 4) Opposite Movement Rule and 5) customized TTFBs®.

The patient must experience the 'cause and effect' of producing their symptoms with their primary aggravating factor (e.g. sustained end range flexion) and then abolishing their symptoms with the corrective action (e.g. posture correction and/or extension movements). This is essential to building musculoskeletal self-efficacy and important to all treatment strategies with the exception of function, where the RSSx do not behave mechanically.

3.   Reduction – this treatment plan is used for patients in the rapid response group that have a relevant loss of joint motion (Stage II – III), and you have proven or strongly expect that the loss can be rapidly eliminated and remain better. These patients are more likely to be seen with acute and subacute disorders; but it is certainly possible with chronic conditions that have clear mechanical behavior of the RSSx. Remember, that most of these patients transitioned through stage 1 and could have been effectively treated with the posture-ergonomic strategy at an earlier point in time.

Phase I – identify procedures that eliminate the relevant loss of motion and control or eliminate the symptoms. This can be achieved in variety of ways, but ultimately must be lasting and functional to have a significant value.

Phase II – this is the process of maintaining the improvements in signs and symptoms until the condition is stabilized (i.e. can no longer be made worse). This can be the most difficult and ultimately the most important phase of the treatment plan. This is achieved through the same basic intervention strategy used for posture-ergonomic (see above) with specific attention to preventing the loss of motion from returning, and specific (quick) reaction when it does.

Phase III – this is the process of reactivating the patient with the intention of returning them to their normal level of activity and function. This recovery of function phase reinforces the importance of balance and activity in the recovery. The ability of the patient to return to normal activity will be the ultimate measurement of the success of the intervention and/or expose the need to progress to a remodeling or stabilization strategy.

Phase   IV – this is the completion of the education and training process for prevention of recurrence. This process began during the initial interview, but is now clarified with regards to long-term instructions for maintenance and service. The patient's knowledge, skills and abilities are tested prior to discharge. We strongly encourage long-term follow-up.

4.   Remodeling – this is the treatment plan for the cumulative response group when there is no evidence of joint instability or nonmechanical behavior. This is most frequently used with chronic disorders and/or patients with longstanding lifestyle factors that are just starting to cause problems. These are stage II or III disorders.

The goal with this patient group is to regain normal motion and/or contraction, and ultimately to restore tolerance to loading and activity. This is the, 'no pain - no gain group'! However, any symptoms that are produced or increased during treatment must not show evidence of causing the condition to deteriorate. This needs to be monitored carefully, especially in the initiation of treatment and when making treatment progressions. All groups are trained in appropriate postural, ergonomic and biomechanical procedures. This can be the strategy from the start of treatment or a progression from another one (e.g. reduction) when it failed to restore the patient to their normal and expected level of activity tolerance. Treatment concludes with individualized prevention training based on the postural-ergonomic strategy.

5.   **Stabilization** – this treatment plan involves exercise and training of the patient to function with optimal body mechanics, maintaining the joint(s) in a mid-range position. The specific strategy is individualized to the patient's condition, ability to control relevant symptoms and signs with TTFB® and functional goals. Therefore, the program may have an extension, lateral, flexion, combination or neutral bias. This is used for structural and functional instabilities that are clinically proven to be relevant.

The program is centered on a progression of strength and conditioning exercises that provide dynamic support to the involved joints and gradually restore the patient's tolerance to load and activity. Therefore it is important to progress this group of patients to therapeutic exercises that are functionally designed to train the patient in proper biomechanical control – this simultaneously provides an assessment of the degree of success of the intervention. This can be the strategy from the start of treatment or a progression from another one (e.g. reduction) when it failed to restore the patient to their normal and expected level of activity tolerance.

6.   **Function** - this treatment plan is used for those patients in the non-mechanical response group. Do not monitor the symptom responses closely. Rather, monitor the response of the signs carefully to insure that the condition is not deteriorating. The intent of the treatment is for the patient to successfully return to work and/or activities; i.e. to regain tolerance to positions, movements and activities. Use the same biomechanical principles as with the postural/ergonomic and stabilization strategies, but without close attention to symptom reporting.

The use of objective measurement tools is very important to the clinical management of this group of patients. Establish a baseline of information regarding pain, perceived function, strength and conditioning. At defined intervals (at least prior to discharge) repeat the same measures and determine the progress. Goals should be set to achieve specific, concrete improvements in physical (functional) capability. This group of patients needs maximal encouragement, and a coordinated, multidisciplinary team approach.

7.   **Other** - this category is for any other treatment plan that does not fall into any of the previous groups.

Table 11-1: Summary Table – The Six DRS Treatment Strategies

Treatment Strategy	General Reasoning	Initial Response Expectations (weeks 1-2)	Outcome Expectations
Anti-inflammatory	Need conservative start; control aggravating factors first to stabilize symptoms; potential to worsen.	Symptoms stable enough to transition – otherwise get help from MD.	If able to transition expectations are based upon the strategy.
Posture-ergonomic	Stage 1 or very early stage 2. All symptoms and any signs easily controlled.	Full Control	Excellent rapid response – long-term is the concern.
Reduction	Stage 2 disorder with loss of rapid control of RSSx	Full control	Excellent rapid response – should be back to full function within 2 – 4 weeks. Long-term is again the concern
Remodeling	Stage 2 or 3 disorder with signs that cannot be rapidly eliminated and/or activity intolerance that cannot be rapidly restored.	Control of symptoms in ADL with p-ergo TTFB® - high rating of recovery does not match change in RSSx and/or function.	Cumulative response; duration to full (potential) recovery or ready for discharge varies with severity ± other factors.
Stabilization	Stage 3 disorder with clinical evidence of joint instability.	Same as remodeling	Same as remodeling
Function	Stage 2 or 3 disorder with non-mechanical behavior of RSSx and disproportionate loss of activity tolerance. Requires clinical paradigm shift.	No significant change – this time period is used for biomechanical training, goal setting & planning.	2 groups: 1) legally involved – RTW is the goal and success is multi-factorial. 2) Not legally involved – cumulative response.

The Reassessment Process

It is easy to examine the patient, come to a conclusion and start a treatment plan. It's another story to see the program through to completion successfully. The success of your intervention is determined in the sequential visits after the initial assessment and treatment, and this is the nitty-gritty of clinical practice. In our system the key to successful treatment is the ongoing and continuous reassessment of the patient's status. This includes readiness to modify or change the plan when needed, willingness to get help, a constructive approach to problem-solving and the need to remain focused to listening to the patient.

The objectives and expectations of the reassessment process are to:

- Determine if your initial conclusions were correct and relevant.
- Determine if the treatment plan is correct and as effective as expected.
- Determine if the patient understands their role in treatment.
- Determine if the patient is performing the techniques properly and effectively.
- Determine if the treatment program needs to be modified or progressed.
- Determine if the treatment plan needs to be changed.
- Determine if the patient is ready for discharge and for the long-term.
- Determine if any inappropriate changes in the patient's condition have occurred.
- Determine the need to refer the patient to a medical physician or specialist.

The components of the reassessment process are as follows:

1.   The reassessment interview – identify how the patient feels they are responding; are there any changes in RSSx they have noted, are there problems implementing the instructions, how active have they been since the last visit etc.?

- **Symptoms** – determine if the location, intensity, frequency and behavior of the symptoms have changed. Correlate any change (better or worse) to the patient's activity level since their last visit.
- **Function/activity** – determine if the patient's ability to tolerate or perform activities, movements, positions has changed. If so how, if not, why not? Compare this to the functional questionnaire ratings.

Be certain to correlate any reported subjective improvements to changes in activity level; this will help you develop a greater understanding of the significance of the changes.

- **Rating of recovery** – the patient is asked to rate the improvement since the initiation of treatment; i.e. the first visit with you. Reassure the patient that any answer is acceptable, and that this is simply a method for communication about how he/she feels they are doing in the treatment program.

0   =   **no improvement whatsoever (or worse)**

100 =   **complete recovery, cured, pain free and function full**

- **Problem identification** – by the end of the interview you should have at least started to isolate the key movements, positions, activities, and time periods of the day in which the patient is having difficulty (if any). You should outline a plan for the patient to fight back against these problems more effectively, and/or pursue further testing or training to address these issues directly (see problem-solving section later in this chapter).

2. Subjective self-management analysis – assess the patient's ability to self-manage. I like to ask the patient to rate their follow through with your instructions using a 0 – 10 scale with the following anchors: 0 = poor, didn't follow through with anything and 10 = excellent, perfect follow through. Compare their ratings to yours and discuss if appropriate.

Self –Efficacy Rating: Poor   0 1 2 3 4 5 6 7 8 9 10   Excellent

In general, you need to determine:

- *Cognition* – do they understand what to do and why to do it?
- *Psychomotor* – do they have the skills to carry-out the plan?
- *Utilization* – do they know how and when to apply this knowledge and skill?

3. Objective self-management analysis – examine the patient's static and dynamic posture, their technique with any self-treatment and/or exercise instruction provided and the response of their RSSx to these procedures. Provide further instruction, change or modification as needed.

4. **Re-examination** – reassess for any change in the patient's relevant signs, give consideration to a more complete reassessment if they are not responding or something has changed in their clinical presentation.

5. **Reassessment conclusions** – after you have completed your reassessment you have enough information to determine the following:

- *Continue the same treatment strategy* – this reassessment conclusion should mean that the patient is gaining, or has gained, full control over RSSX and they are progressing towards achievement of functional goals with the current strategy. The patient's recovery rating(s) should be continuously improving with supportive evidence of improvement in the RSSx and/or function. The idea is not to change something that is working; wait and see if the current strategy is all that is required to solve their problem – but be prepared to progress or modify the plan if they hit a plateau.
- *Progress/modify the same treatment strategy* – this reassessment conclusion indicates that the patient has hit a plateau, or is not responding as well as expected and you need to find a better way to gain control over the RSSx and improve function. This includes progressing manual therapy procedures, use of various mechanical devices (traction, braces etc.), therapeutic exercise, various modalities etc. How you progress or modify the treatment strategy depends on the initial strategy chosen, but the bottom-line is that the plan needs to be adjusted to keep the patient moving towards full recovery or maximum benefit.
- *Retest to change to a new treatment strategy* – this reassessment conclusion is reserved for when the patient is just not responding well at all (i.e. no improvement or reporting to be worse). This could be due to an incorrect initial conclusion, or something has changed. Wipe the slate clean, and reassess to see if you need to change your conclusions, change your treatment plan or seek help from the referring physician, specialist or a more experienced colleague.
- *Add New Treatment Strategy* – this reassessment conclusion indicates that the current treatment plan has helped, but only to a limited degree. So reassess the patient to see if you need to change

the emphasis of the program. This always occurs with the anti-inflammatory strategy as it is a transitional plan. Another example is when the patient initially demonstrated an ability to improve rapidly, but control over the RSSx with the existing strategy is inadequate to restore activity tolerance and achieve the functional goals. A common change of treatment strategy would be to initiate a remodeling or stabilization strategy when you are having difficulty achieving the functional goals. However any change is possible depending upon the response of the patient.

Clinical Problem-solving

The following comments about problem-solving assume that contraindications have been ruled out and cautions identified and appropriately addressed. Our motto is; *"The presence of a problem is the opportunity for a solution!"*

One example of needing to implement problem-solving techniques is when the patient reports a 'flare-up' of their condition. The key to sorting this out is to isolate the critical factors that caused the flare-up, then find and implement a specific solution. This is a great opportunity to build the patient's musculoskeletal self-efficacy; stimulated by proven 'cause and effect' control over the RSSx (see table 11-2). This problem-solving process starts with the following:

- *Time* – when (exactly) did the problem in controlling the RSSx develop?
- *Place* – where was the patient when this occurred and what were they doing?
- *Response* – what did the patient do in response to the return/increase of the RSSx and when did they do it?
- *Other* – are there any other relevant factors?
- *Conclusions* – based on the information obtained, isolate the source of the problem and formulate and prioritize potential solutions.
- *Plan* – implement solutions in a logical sequence based on your prioritization until you find a solution and/or are forced back to the 'drawing board'.

Flare-up	Most Likely Cause	Most Likely Solution
Woke with an increase of pain.	Slept in a position that strained the musculoskeletal structure or tissue.	Change the sleeping position, surface and/or provide supports or pillows.
Increase of pain upon performing the TTFB®	Technique is performed incorrectly or not adjusted to a change in RSSx.	Correct or modify the technique – prove what is correct.
During day performing sedentary work/ ADL	Lost biomechanical control and/or in static load for too long.	Correct posture and/or ergonomics; adjust frequency of micro-pauses and OMR stretches.
During day performing light to medium demanding work/ADL	Lost biomechanical control, fatigue and/or did not use TTFB® proactively or with quick reaction to warning signals.	Correct posture, body mechanics and use of TTFB® (including checking technique and effectiveness). In addition may need strategic strength and conditioning.
During day performing heavy demanding work/ADL	Same as light to medium work/ADL.	Same with greater likelihood of needing strategic strength and conditioning to ultimately control the problem.
At end of day, after work and activities	Loss of biomechanical control and/or in static load too long when relaxing prior to going to sleep.	Correct posture and/or biomechanics; use TTFB® more effectively; be more active prior to sleeping.

Table 11-2: Examples of possible causes of flare-up with the most likely solutions; assuming you have 'sorted-out' the source through a disciplined, problem-solving process.

Problem-solving is also required when a patient fails to improve, hits a plateau in their recovery, or reports to be worsening. This was covered in the reassessment section, but can be summarized as follows:

1.   There is no subjective or objective improvement – the basic presumptions are that your conclusions and/or treatment strategy is incorrect, or the patient is not implementing the self-management procedures effectively. The patient's self-treatment skills, knowledge and application of their TTFB® system needs to be directly assessed – if the TTFB® procedures are effective in the clinic you need to spend more time training the patient. If they are not effective (i.e. which means that they are not TTFB® by definition) you need to carefully re-evaluate to determine if relevant findings were overlooked, the treatment strategy needs to be changed or modified. Possibilities include that your initial conclusions were incorrect or you did not recognize multiple disorders presenting simultaneously.

2.   Improvements have stalled – the basic presumptions are that the treatment strategy needs to be progressed, modified or changed. This requires careful analysis that includes the following general possibilities:

- If the RSSx are consistently eliminated or controlled by the TTFB® procedures, but keep returning, then focus on identifying what triggers the recurrence and place more emphasis on biomechanical control, proactive interruption of the activity with the TTFB® ± need for strategic strength and conditioning if physical demands issues are relevant.
- In the case of the reduction strategy, if the motion loss is not fully eliminated and/or the improvements do not remain better under load then the progression of force concept is indicated. Manual or mechanical procedures need to be explored further. This same concept applies to the remodeling strategy; e.g. a need to increase intensity and/or frequency of stretching, or employ the progressive TFM concept etc. Additionally, there is always the possible need for strategic strength and conditioning if physical demands issues are relevant and you have not progressed to this phase of treatment.
- You may have hit the maximum benefit of the initial treatment strategy and you now need to transition to another. A classic example is when a reduction strategy fails to restore the patient's tolerance to weight bearing with low back derangement syndromes in a reasonable timeframe; the treatment needs to transition to stabilization or remodeling.
- You may have overlooked another symptom-generator (i.e. there are multiple disorders) in which case you need to reassess and identify the distinguishing patterns of response and methods for control.
- There may be a comorbidity that requires attention, including consultation with the medical practitioner; e.g. side effect of a medication etc.

3. **Patient reports to be worsening** – when the patient reports to be worsening, and especially if there is evidence that their RSSx have deteriorated and/or new signs and symptoms have emerged that are nonmechanical, you need to refer to medical physician (see chapter on cautions and contraindications). Should the patient be fully 'worked-up' and there are no clear contraindications to treatment, yet they continue to report to be worsening, your approach is not working – get help from

a colleague, consult the other members of the healthcare team and/or refer to someone that you know has more experience or special skills relevant to the patient's problem.

Summary

Successful treatment is dependent on a number of factors, some of which are within our control and others that are not. Simply because a patient gets better does not mean your treatment was effective. You need to establish a 'cause and effect' control over the patient's RSSx, evaluate the response in light of natural history, return the patient to full function and ultimately evaluate the long-term impact.

This chapter presented the six treatment strategies utilized in our system in an attempt to successfully manage the widest cross-section of ARMSD possible. We stressed the importance of having a structured and continuous reassessment process to optimize results and recognize when and why to get help. An introduction to basic problem-solving techniques was provided to help clinicians overcome common barriers to patient recovery.

References Chapter 11

Abenhaim L, Rossignol M, Valat JP, et al. The role of activity in the therapeutic management of back pain: report of the international Paris task force on back pain. Spine 25 (4S): 1S – 33S, 2000.

Bandura, A. Self-efficacy: The exercise of control. WH Freeman and Co., New York, 1997.

Edwards RR, Almeida DM, Klick B, Haythornwaite JA, Smith MT. Duration of sleep contributes to next-day pain report in the general population. Pain 137 (1): 202-7, 2008.

Hubble MA, Duncan BL, Miller SD. The Heart & Soul of Change: What Works in Therapy. American Psychological Association, Washington D.C., 1999.

Karas R, McIntosh G, Hall H, et al. The relationship between nonorganic signs and centralization of symptoms in the prediction of return to work for patients with low back pain. Phys Ther 77:354–60, 1997.

Marin R, Cyhan T, Miklos W: Sleep disturbance in patients with chronic low back pain. Am J Phys Med Rehabil 85:430-435, 2006.

Neck Pain Task Force: The Bone and Joint Decade (2000-2010) Task Force on Neck Pain and Its Associated Disorders. Spine 33 (4S): S1 – S220, 2008

Rath W. Cervical traction: a clinical perspective. Orthopaedic Review, 13(8), 29-48, 1984.

Rath W. Meeting the healthcare challenge: the marriage of quality and cost. McKenzie Institute Newsletter 2(2): 3 – 5, 1994.

Rath W. Case study-patient evaluation and treatment (Nancy). McKenzie Institute Newsletter, US. 3(2): 50 - 53, 1995.

Rath W. Outcome assessment in clinical practice. The McKenzie Institute Journal. 4(3): 9-16, 1996.

Rath W. Clinical practice: it is both art and science. The McKenzie Journal 6(1): 5, 1998.

Rath W, Rath JD. Outcome assessment in clinical practice. The McKenzie Journal 6(2): 17-20, 1998.

Rath JD, Rath W, Mielcarsky E, Waldman R. Low back pain in pregnancy: helping patients take control. The Journal of Musculoskeletal Medicine. 17 (4): 223 –232, 2000.

Rath W. Spinal Manipulative Therapy and the Prevention of Dysfunction and Disability. Combined Sections Meeting, Orthopaedic Section, APTA, Boston, MA, Feb. 23, 2002.

Werneke MW, Hart DL, Resnik L, Stratford PW, Reyes A. Centralization: prevalence and effect on treatment outcomes using a standardized operational definition and measurement method. JOSPT 38 (3):116-25, 2008.

Chapter 12: Planning for the Long-term

The patient experience can be a turning point in their lives. On one hand it can be the start of a life of chronic pain, impairment and disability; or it can mark the beginning of an active and healthy life that carries into retirement and beyond. Why and how either happens is multifactorial, but the influence of the attitude, beliefs and the approach of the care-givers is significant. In regards to musculoskeletal disorders, iatrogenesis is a growing problem (Abenheim 1995; Flynn 2011; Pransky 2011).

It is important to have a long-term view when treating patients for a number of reasons; some of these are expressed in the 2nd edition of the "Burden of Musculoskeletal Diseases in the United States" (Jacobs 2011): By 2030 the number of people over age of 65 is projected to double, with aged 85 and over the most rapidly expanding segment of society. Incidence of MSD and resulting disability increases with aging: on an age-adjusted basis MSD are reported by 48% of the population (compared to 30% circulatory and 24% respiratory). At the age > 75 years there is a 69% incidence of MSD and 74% for circulatory (this includes coronary and heart conditions). MSD are the number one cause of limited ADL (back pain the most likely cause); twofold greater than the next category (circulatory). Chronic joint pain peaks in the 65 – 74 year age group; knee and shoulder joint pain problems are most common.

Of course it is also possible that the patient experience has no long-term influence; i.e. a non-effect. This is a lost opportunity, especially with the tendency for most MSD to be recurrent and there are many other beneficial health effects of enhancing musculoskeletal self-efficacy. There is an abundance of evidence now that remaining active is critical to lifelong health (Booth 2000, 2002; Manson 2002; Myers 2002; Byberg 2009; Pate 2010; Sun 2010). MSDs are often the initial cause of limited activity that gradually cascades into a series of health problems and other morbidities.

Interactive Treatment

Planning for discharge should commence at the initial assessment and treatment session. The basic information and skills the patient needs to prevent recurrence of the same MSD should be developed during the course of their care and not left to the last session. In addition to preparing the patient for the long-term, a patient who is actively involved in their recovery usually recovers more quickly. The interaction of the therapist with the patient while identifying and explaining the RSSx, searching for TTFBs® (i.e. procedures during which the patient experiences the cause and effect of controlling their RSSx), and while planning how to achieve functional goals, are key elements to habit change and musculoskeletal self-efficacy.

The late Wilbert Fordyce (1976) was one of the first to understand the importance of the biopsychosocial model and its application to successful treatment of chronic musculoskeletal pain and disability – his was a behavioral approach that remains effective and applicable today (Butler 2010). In response to a research article in Spine he made the following comment about treating back pain in primary practice that has great applicability; "A mindset of coach rather than repairman should be adopted in the general attitude and social posture taken toward the patient" (Fordyce 1996).

This is an important change in mindset for many clinicians, as most of us want to figure out the patient's problem and then do something that 'fixes' them. But, can you really 'fix' a disorder that is generated by habits, has a strong tendency to recur, and one in which successful treatment is (ultimately) measured by an ability to remain active for a lifetime? We can apply techniques that have a specific and immediate effect on RSSx, but preserving activity tolerance for the long-term is up to the patient. That requires the mindset of a coach, and an approach that encourages the patient to make a change.

Self-determination theory has identified that the best methods to achieve a positive change in health behaviors is to provide the patient with a compelling reason, and incorporate an approach that encourages them to integrate actions that lead to new behaviors (Deci 2002; Williams 2002). Habit change research demonstrates the importance of repetition of actions linked to achieving specific goals as a key to effecting change (Markland 2005; Neal 2006; Nicholas 2007; Wood 2005; 2007). Getting patients to change habits and behavior is a major challenge in healthcare, but essential to a prevention-based paradigm (see table 12-1).

Table 12-1: Self-determination theory (SDT) and new perspectives in habit change research are relevant to using the patient experience as a tool to achieve a long-term effect. The following provides a brief 'sound-bite' of these areas of research.	
Self-Determination Theory	**Habit Change Research**
3 Innate Psychological needs: competence, autonomy and relatedness. Individuals are proactive and engaged or passive and alienated – mostly a function of social conditions during development and function. SDT is focused to social-contextual conditions that facilitate self-motivation and healthy psychological function (Deci 2000).	Habits are products of gradual learning of association between responses and performance contexts. Goals can direct habits by motivating the repetition to change that is required and exposure to cues that reinforce the habit and preserve the habit that can lead to self-regulation (Wood 2007).

Transition to Self-management (Discharge)

The transition to self-management formally occurs when the patient is discharged from treatment having achieved a maximal benefit. The point of maximal benefit is easy to determine when the outcome is either great (i.e. clearly no further need) or poor (i.e. hasn't responded positively at all). It's when the patient improves partially that it can be difficult to recognize maximal benefit and time for discharge. This is a decision that the clinician and patient should make together rather than being made by the third party payer. There are several keys to improving your recognition that the patient is ready even though they have not fully recovered:

1. Appropriate objective measurements demonstrate that progress has plateaued in spite of attempts to change/progress treatment for a sustained time period.

2. The patient has been on program for an adequate time period (e.g.

at least an average number of weeks and visits for the musculoskeletal region and disorder with consideration to comorbidities).

3.   You have confidence that the particular MSD will resolve over time (i.e. natural history) provided the patient remains active.

4.   The patient has a path to full achievement of function goals, and the treatment program has been activity-oriented with a long-term plan.

5. The patient agrees to the discharge plan and there are arrangements for long-term follow-up and problem-solving if needed.

Provide the patient with written and/or electronic instructions for reference, reminders and simple problem-solving relevant to their individual problem. Review the 5 core elements as they apply to the individual patient and their treatment plan. Do some sort of follow-up; you might be surprised how well most of your patients are doing, especially the ones who had to struggle to achieve improvements.

Outcome Assessment ("Internal Evidence")

The Duffy-Rath System© is dedicated to ongoing analysis of its interventions and to supporting clinical research at all levels of scientific scrutiny. Having a system to objectively assess the response of your patients to the care you provided is the basis for the 'Internal Evidence' we discussed in earlier sections of the workshop – this is the most important evidence for your practice. External evidence meets high levels of scientific standards, is generalizable and important for designing your programs, procedures and strategies – but how the patient actually responds in your hands is ultimately more important. In patient care, internal evidence trumps external evidence.

There are four basic steps to ongoing outcome assessment in clinical practice:

1.   Initial data collection: identify and operationalize the independent and dependent variables you are going to track and compare; collect baseline measures.

2. Ongoing data collection: track relevant changes in key measures, identify any changes to treatment, conditions etc. that could impact analysis and/or outcome.

3) Final data collection: repeat all measures taken at baseline that are required for outcome assessment, plus any additional measures that are appropriate (e.g. satisfaction survey etc.).

4) Follow-up data collection: repeat key measures at certain time periods after discharge to assess any long-term effects.

General Outcomes to be Measured (Dependent Variables):

- **Clinical Effectiveness:** this is measured by the amount of improvement in the key measures (i.e. dependent variables). Our system assesses improvement in pain and functional ratings, the patient rating of recovery, change in RSSx and return to work status when applicable.
- **Clinical Efficiency:** this is measured by the number of treatment sessions (visits) and weeks compared to a standard and/or natural history.
- **Cost of Service:** this includes total charges for physical therapy services; total healthcare services when applicable and available; and the relative worth or value of the time and effort spent by patient and therapist in achieving the eventual outcome (i.e. behavioral accounting).
- **Satisfaction:** measurement of the patient's satisfaction with the clinical and office service as determined by a questionnaire.
- **Follow-up:** this is determined by phone, mail or internet survey, or a follow-up visit.

Duffy-Rath Outcome Rankings

Since 1985 we have tracked outcomes for patient treatment; with six categories of response: 1) excellent, 2) good, 3) fair, 4) poor, 5) unknown, 6) not applicable (see table 12-2). These outcomes are determined by comparing the status of the patient at the initial assessment and treatment visit to the last visit or documented evidence of patient response (this can be a documented follow-up phone call or email etc.), as follows:

Table 12-2: the DRS definitions of outcome categories.
Excellent – the patient has achieved full control over RSSx, is fully active (i.e. if they were idle, they have returned to work, and function goals have been achieved), rates 90 % recovery or greater, all VAS ratings of pain and disability are less than 2.
Good – the patient has achieved full control over RSSx, is fully active (i.e. if they were idle, they have returned to work, but this may be to restricted duty, and function goals have been achieved), rates 70 % recovery or greater, all VAS ratings of pain and disability are less than 5 (unless the response group was non-mechanical. In this case the VAS ratings had to improve, but do not need to be all less than 5).
Fair – there has been measured improvement in some or all of the criteria, but not enough to be placed into the good category.
Poor – the patient demonstrated no improvement in any subjective, objective or functional measurements.
Unknown – the patient dropped-out so the outcome to treatment is not known, and there is not enough data or enough visits to identify a category. As a general rule, any patient seen for 4 or more visits has to have an outcome.
Not Applicable – the intent of physical therapy was not to treat (consultation or a structured evaluation like an FCE, etc.).

Patient Satisfaction – we collect information about patient satisfaction with the care they received by survey using 5 possible ratings: 2 are positive (1 strongly and the other moderately), 2 negative (1 strongly and the other moderately) and 1 neutral – the following operational definitions must be followed in determining the category of outcome (see table 12-3). Deyo (1998) and Hurwitz (2005) recognize the 'stand-alone' importance of patient satisfaction as a powerful measure of outcome.

Table 12-3: definitions of DRS satisfaction ratings.
Excellent – all questions are answered with the highest possible rating of satisfaction.
Good – all questions are answered with a positive response, but not all are the highest possible rating.
Fair – there is a mixture of positive and negative responses.
Poor – all responses are negative.
Unknown – the survey was not completed, or the patient indicates no opinion for the questions.

Minimally Important Change

How much improvement is needed to demonstrate a clinical benefit is a debatable and variable subject (van Tuder 2007; Kho 2009; Wilson 2011) – however there are standards that can be useful (Ostello 2008) as illustrated in the following; table 12-4:

Table 12-4: Ostello et. al. (2008) proposed guidelines for minimal important change (MIC) with scores of pain and functional status.			
Questionnaire	Scoring Range	MIC (absolute cutoff)	MIC (% improvement from baseline)
VAS	0 – 100	15	30
NRS	0 – 10	2	30
Roland Disability	0 – 24	5	30
Oswestry Disability	0 – 100	10	30
Quebec Back Pain Disability	0 – 100	20	30

Factors that can Affect Outcome

The following is an overview of the general effect that certain factors have had on outcomes in each of our clinics since 1985 (see table 12-5). This information should be used to improve your clinical management strategies; however this is not randomized, controlled research data - generalizations cannot (and should not) be made.

Table 12-5: Factors That Influence Treatment Response: the expected response is 85 - 90 % Good/Excellent Outcome, Average of 6 visits (±2), over a period of 4 – 5 weeks (±2).		
Independent Variable	Outcome	Utilization
Symptom Location	No significant effect	No significant effect
Symptom Duration	No significant effect when excellent/ good outcomes are combined. Acute/subacute have more excellent outcomes than chronic.	Chronic disorders require more visits and weeks on program to achieve good/excellent outcome
Neurologic Signs	Decreased excellent/good outcomes when present and relevant.	Patients with MSD with relevant neurologic signs require more visits and weeks on program to achieve fair/good/excellent outcome.
Activity Status	Working/active patients have an increased likelihood of an excellent/ good outcome.	Idle/inactive patients require more visits and weeks on program to achieve good/excellent outcome.
Adverse Behavioral Signs & Symptoms	Decreased excellent/good outcomes when present.	Patients with relevant behavioral signs & symptoms require more visits and weeks on program to achieve fair/good/excellent outcome. Continued next page

| Spinal Region | No significant effect. | Thoracic responds the quickest, followed by cervical, then lumbo-sacral, and last was combination disorders. |
| Litigation Relevant to MSD | Decreased excellent/good outcomes when present. | Patients with relevant litigation require more visits and weeks on program to achieve fair/good/ excellent outcomes. |

It is always important to determine if a treatment approach is replicable; i.e. can others achieve the same or similar results. The following table overviews the results of a consecutive case series involving 7 physical therapists who completed the DRS certification course (see table 12-6).

Effectiveness and efficiency was very similar to our findings; fair outcomes did reach the standard for minimally important change; poor outcomes had the least number of visits and weeks, while the longer the patient was on program the greater their chance of a good outcome. This last finding is extremely important to defend the appropriateness of our service and the need for more visits and time when required.

Table 12-6: Preliminary report of outcome findings with a consecutive case-series investigation (N = 166) with 7 clinicians completing the Duffy-Rath certification system (Rath et. al. 2008 – unpublished data).

Outcome Category	NRS IE	NRS DC	DRQ IE	DRQ DC	Visits	Weeks
Excellent N = 65; 39.2 %	4.97	0.3	40.0	5.8	6.6	4.1
Good N = 54; 32.5 %	5.9	1.7	46.9	15.6	7.3	4.4
Fair N = 39; 23.5 %	5.7	3.7	56.4	41.8	9.0	5.0
Poor N = 8; 4.8 %	4.8	6.0	55.7	58.2	4.9	3.1

Summary

Our mission statement summarizes our approach to MSDs; "Our mission is the prevention of musculoskeletal and lifestyle-related disorders and disability through education, training and research." In our approach treatment of MSDs is a secondary and tertiary prevention activity. Whatever approach you adopt in clinical practice we strongly encourage that you develop methods to get the patient actively involved in their care and focused to their long-term health and function. Now that you are familiar with this introductory material you have a solid basis for learning our approach to regional MSD; i.e. the back, neck, upper limb, lower limb and chronic musculoskeletal pain and disability.

References Chapter 12

Abenhaim L, Rossignol M, Valat JP, et al. The role of activity in the therapeutic management of back pain: report of the international Paris task force on back pain. Spine 25 (4S): 1S – 33S, 2000.

Bandura, A. Self-efficacy: The exercise of control. WH Freeman and Co., New York, 1997.

Booth FW, Gordon SE, Carlson CJ, Hamilton MT. Waging war on modern chronic diseases: primary prevention through exercise biology. Journal Applied Physiology 88: 774-87, 2000.

Booth FW, Chakravarthy MV, Gordon SE, Spangenburg EE.Waging war on physical inactivity: using modern molecular ammunition against an ancient enemy. J Applied Physiology 93: 3 – 30, 2002.

Byberg L, Melhus H, Gedeborg R, et. al. Total mortality after changes in leisure time physical activity in 50 year old men: 35 year follow-up of population based cohort. British Medical Journal (BMJ 2009; 338;b688 doi:10.1136/bmj.b688)

Butler S. A personal experience learning from two pain pioneers, JJ Bonica and W Fordyce: lessons surviving four decades of pain practice. Scand J Pain 1 (1): 34-37, 2010.

Deci EL, Ryan RM. Self-determination theory and the facilitation of intrinsic motivation, social development, and well-being. American Psychologist 55 (1): 68-78, 2000.

Deci EL, Ryan RM, Editors. Handbook of Self-Determination Research. University of Rochester Press, Rochester, NY, 2002.

Deyo RA, Battié M, Beurskens AJHM, et. al. Outcome measures for low back pain research: a proposal for standardized use. Spine 23 (18): 2003-13, 1998.

Flynn TW, Smith B, Chou R. Appropriate use of diagnostic imaging in low back pain: a reminder that unnecessary imaging may do as much harm as good. JOSPT 41 (11): 838-46, 2011.

Fordyce WE: Behavioral Methods in Chronic Pain and Illness.St. Louis: CV Mosby; 1976.

Fordyce WE. Point of view: educational and behavioral interventions for back pain in primary care. Spine 21 (24): 2858 – 59, 1996.

Hurwitz EL, Morgenstern H, Yu F. Satisfaction as a Predictor of Clinical Outcomes Among Chiropractic and Medical Patients Enrolled in the UCLA Low Back Pain Study. Spine. 30(19):2121-2128, 2005.

Jacobs JJ (Chair, Management Oversight Team). The Burden of Musculoskeletal Diseases in the United States, 2nd Edition. Rosemont, IL 2011.

Kho ME, Duffett M, Willison DJ, Cook DJ, Brouwers MC. Written informed consent and selection bias in observational studies using medical records: systematic review. BMJ 2009; 338:b866 doi:10.1136/bmj.b866.

Krismer M, van Tulder M. The low back pain group of the bone and joint health strategies European project. Best Prac Res Clin Rheumatol 21 (1): 77-91, 2007

Manson JE, Greenland P, LaCroix AZ, et. al. Walking compared with vigorus exercise for the prevention of cardiovascular events in woman. New England Journal of Medicine 347 (10); 716 -25, 2002.

Markland D, Ryan RM, Tobin VJ, Rollnick S. Motivational interviewing and self-determination theory. J Social Clinical Psychology 24 (6): 811-31, 2005.

Morken T, Mageroy N, Moen BE. Physical activity is associated with a low prevalence of musculoskeletal disorders in the Royal Norwegian navy: a cross sectional study. BMC Musculoskeletal Disorders 2007, 8:56 doi:10.1186/1471-24748-56

Myers J, Prakash M, Froelicher V, Do D, Partington S, Atwood JE. Exercise capacity and mortality among men referred for exercise testing. New England Journal Medicine 346 (11): 793 – 801, 2002.

National Center for Health Statistics. Health, United States, 2010: With Special Feature on Death and Dying. Hyattsville, MD. 2011 (http://www.cdc.gov/nchs/data/hus/hus10.pdf)

Neal DT, Wood W, Quinn JM. Habits-a repeat performance. Curr Dir Psychol Sci 15 (4): 198-202, 2006.

Pate RR, Yancey AK, Kraus WE. The 2008 Physical Activity Guidelines for Americans: implications for clinical and public health practice. American Journal of Lifestyle Medicine 4 (3): 209-17, 2010.

Pransky G, Borkan JM, Young AE, Cherkin DC. Are we making progress? The tenth international forum for primary care research on low back pain. Spine 36 (19): 1608-14, 2011.

Rath JD, Rath W, Mielcarsky E, Waldman R. Low back pain in pregnancy: helping patients take control. The Journal of Musculoskeletal Medicine April; 223 –232, 2000.

Soukup MG, Glomsröd B, Lönn JH, Bö K, Larsen S, Fordyce WE. The Effect of a Mensendieck Exercise Program as Secondary Prophylaxis for Recurrent Low Back Pain A Randomized, Controlled Trial With 12-Month Follow-up Spine 1999;24:1585

Sun Q, Townsend MK, Okereke OI, et. al. Physical activity at midlife in relation to successful survival in women at age 70 years or older. Archives Internal Medicine 170 (2): 194-201, 2010.

van Tulder M, Malmivaara A, Hayden J, Koes B. Statistical significance versus clinical importance. Spine 32 (16): 1785-90, 2007.

Wand BM, Bird C, McAuley JH, Dore CJ, MacDowell M, DeSouza LH. Early intervention for the management of acute low back pain: a single-blind randomized controlled trial of biopsychosocial education, manual therapy and exercise. Spine 29 (21): 2350-56, 2004.

Weber H: The natural history of disc herniation and the influence of intervention. Spine 19 (19): 2234-2238, 1994.

Werneke M, Hart D. Centralization Phenomenon as a Prognostic Factor for Chronic Low Back Pain and Disability. Spine.26(7):758-764,2001.

Williams GC. Improving patient's health through supporting autonomy of patients and providers. IN: Deci EL, Ryan RM, ed. Handbook of Self-determination Research. University of Rochester Press, Rochester, NY, 2002: pp 233-54.

Wilson HD, Mayer TG, Gatchel RJ. The lack of association between changes in functional outcomes and work retention in a chronic disabling occupational spinal disorder population. Spine 36 (6): 474 – 80, 2011.

Wood W, Neal DT. A new look at habits and the habit-goal interface. Psych Rev 114 (4): 843 – 63, 2007.

Woolf AD, Pfleger B. Burden of major musculoskeletal conditions. Bulletin of the WHO 81 (9): 646-56, 2003.

List of DRS Abbreviations in Alphabetical Order

Abbreviation	Definition
A	Abolish(es)
ACC	Accident Compensation Commission (New Zealand)
ACJ	Acromioclavicular Joint
ADL	Activities of Daily Living
APTA	American Physical Therapy Association
AROM	Active range of motion
ARSD	Activity-related spinal disorder
B	Better
BPS	BioPsychoSocial
C	Centralization
CCR	Canadian C-spine Rule
CDC	Centers for Disease Control
CE1	Core Element 1 (Biomechanical Control)
CE2	Core Element 2 (Effectively manage fatigue & warning signals)
CE3	Core Element 3 (Healthy or adequate range of motion)
CE4	Core Element 4 Strategic strength and conditioning)
CE5	Core Element 5 (Positve attitude for musculoskeletal self-efficacy)
CI	Confidence Interval
CIC	Carpal instability complex
CID	Carpal instability dissociative
CIND	Carpal instability nondissociative
CP	Centralization Phenomenon
CPR	Clinical Prediction Rule
CPT	Combined Performance Technique
CRPS	Complex Regional Pain Syndrome
D or ↓	Decrease(s)
DF	Degrees of Freedom
DM	During movement
DP	Directional Preference
DRQ	Duffy-Rath Questionnaire
DRS	Duffy-Rath System©

E	Excellent
ER	End range (grade 2 mobilization)
ER	End range
EROP	End range overpressure (grade 3 mobilization)
F	Fair
FNS	Femoral Nerve Stretch
G	Good
GCS	Glasgow Coma Scale
GHJ	Glenohumeral Joint
HHS	Health and Human Services
HI	Hypothenar ischial (spinal manipulation technique)
I or ↑	Increase(s)
IASP	International Association for the Study of Pain
ICC	Intraclass coefficient
ICF	International Classification of Functioning, Disability and Health
ISQ	In Status Quo
ISSLS	International Society for the Study of the Lumbar Spine
k	Kappa coefficient
LBP	Low back pain
LLL	Long lever lumbar (spinal manipulation technique)
LR	Likelihood Ratio
MIC	Minimmally important change
MMPI	Minnesota Multiphasic Personality Inventory
MMT	Manual Muscle Testing
MP	Mammillary push (spinal manipulation technique)
MR	Mid-range (grade 1 mobilization)
MSD	Muculoskeletal Disorder
MT	Manual Therapy
MWM	Mobilization with Movement (Mulligan)
N	Newton (NM = newton meter)
NA	Not applicable
NAG	Mulligan PA Mobilization of Neck and Upper Back Sitting
NASS	North American Spine Society
NB	No Better
NE	No Effect

NIE	No Incident or Event
NLC	NEXUS low risk criteria (for blunt trauma to neck)
NPI	Neck Pain Index
NPV	Negative Predictive Value
NRS	Numeric Rating Scale
NW	No Worse
O	Other
ODI	Oswestry Disability Index
OR	Odds ratio
OST	Orthopaedic Specialty Test
P	Poor
PDM	Pain during movement
PER	Pain end range
PPV	Positive Predictive Value
PRISMA	Preferred Reporting Items for Systematic Reviews and Meta-Analysis
PROM	Passive range of motion
PTFMR	Positive TFM Response
QTF	Quebec Task Force
QTF1	Local spine pain only
QTF2	Local spine pain + proximal limb
QTF3	Local spine pain + distal limb (BK or BE)
QTF4	Radiculopathy
QTFR	Quebec Task Force Report
RMDQ	Roland Morris Disability Questionnaire
ROM	Range of Motion
RROM	Resisted range of motion
RS/CTD	Repetitive Strain/Cumulative Trauma Disorder
RSSx	Relevant Signs and Symptoms
RTW	Return To Work
S/P	Status post
SCJ	Sternoclavicular Joint
SDT	Self-determination Theory
SLR	Straight Leg Raise
SMT	Spinal Manual (Manipulative) Therapy
SNAG	Sustained Natural Apopyseal Glide (Mulligan Neck MWM)

Stage 1	Warning signal stage
Stage 2	Nonspecific disorder stage
Stage 3	Structural pathology Stage
STARD	Standards for the Reporting of Diagnostic Accuracy Studies
STROBE	Strengthening the Reporting of Observational Studies in Epidemiology
TFCC	Triangular Fibrocartilage Complex (Ulnar wrist)
TFM	Transverse Friction Massage
TTFB®	Tools To Fight Back®
UK	Unknown
ULT	Upper Limb Tension
ULTT	Upper Limb Tension Test
VAS	Visual Analogue Scale
VAS	Varies
VBI	Vertebro-Basilar Insufficiency
W	Worse
WAD	Whiplash Associated Disorder
WHO	World Health Organization
WLC	Work-Life-Conflict
WRMSD	Work-related MSD

WAYNE RATH & JEAN DUFFY RATH

Wayne and Jean are owners of Duffy-Rath Physical Therapy, PC and founders of the Duffy-Rath System© for the prevention of activity-related musculoskeletal disorders; e.g. back and neck pain, shoulder impingement, carpal tunnel, degenerative joint disorders etc. They have pioneered a unique, evidence-based approach to these common problems since 1984, and have had a major influence on the diagnosis, treatment and prevention of spine pain and cumulative musculoskeletal disorders internationally.

Their mission is: "The prevention of musculoskeletal and lifestyle-related disorders and disability through education, training and research". Application of their system provides individuals with knowledge, skills and confidence to control their biomechanical health and ability; "Tools To Fight Back®" that guide people to staying active through their working years and into retirement.

Jean is the Director of prevention services, and Wayne directs treatment, continuing education and research. They have many prevention programs ongoing throughout the United States with continuous expansion based on word of mouth marketing.

Workshops are provided to train healthcare professionals, company management and safety professionals, workers and the general public about their system. This introductory book is for healthcare clinicians and is the first in a series. It provides a baseline of knowledge, information and perspective needed to learn clinical application of the system.

For more information go to: www.duffyrath.com.

www.ingramcontent.com/pod-product-compliance
Lightning Source LLC
Chambersburg PA
CBHW061739270326
41928CB00011B/2298